PRAISE FC

Cravings

Former Cosmo bureau chief Wanda Hennig charts her search for freedom, great sex and herself through food, Zen and orgasmic meditation. —*Cosmopolitan*

◯

Zen-inspiration rescues memoirist Wanda Hennig, a one-time contributor to this magazine, who shares her inner turmoil: deep depression, binge eating and severe social anxiety. Pick up the paperback to be instantly transported from Paris and Pocatello to South Africa and San Francisco. —*Alameda Magazine*

◯

In this thoughtful and teasing memoir, Durban-born writer Wanda Hennig chronicles her lively desire to explore overseas destinations in geographic, gourmand and even erotic terms. Elegantly witty. —*Farmer's Weekly*

◯

Hennig has a university background in psychology. Add to this the Zen experience and her branching out into life coaching— in America as well as South Africa—and one appreciates the background that made this book possible. —*The Mercury*

◯

Hennig leaves behind boyfriends, a dog, and even a daughter on her journey to find herself. Ultimately, she does with a lot of Zen meditation fueling her sensual spin halfway around the world in an everyday existence filled with sexuality that drives her ever-present "Wanda-lust." —*Oakland Magazine*

Wanda Hennig's sensitive, engaging and honest memoir is a highly personal, readable and unusual book. It is also very funny and captures life and its meaning without once sounding like some kind of lecture. Several years in a Zen Buddhist temple—the teachings and contemplations—assist the author in her discovery of her true self. Hennig shrinks from nothing, not even some of the bizarre sexual therapy on offer in California. —*Independent Newspapers*

Cravings has been described as a compelling, gritty, courageously honest, page-turning account of one person's life facing her demons, punctuated by lessons in Zen practice, devoid of mystery and esoteric philosophy; and as a fun, trippy book about an intimate subject. —*Sunday Tribune*

It seems unlikely to use the words "nymphonosher" and Buddhist teacher in the same breath when describing a person. Yet author Wanda Hennig is a complex mix of both. Having had a tumultuous relationship with food in her twenties, Hennig, who has post-graduate degrees in psychology and education, takes a long hard look at food, love and sex and how they can become a toxic mix. "Do not deprive yourself, fall in love with food and eat sensually. Enjoy the challenge, pleasure and adventure of each moment," she tells readers in *Cravings*. —*Saturday Independent*

Cravings

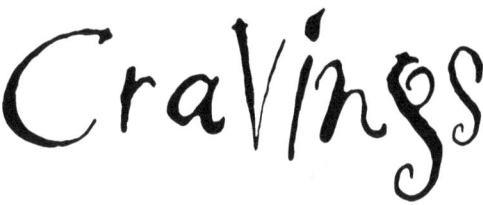

A Zen-inspired memoir
about sensual pleasures, freedom from
dark places, and living and eating
with abandon

WANDA HENNIG

Say
Yes
Press

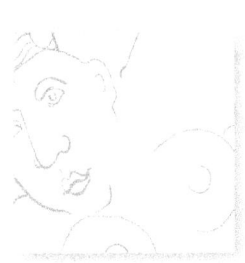

First published in paperback and eBook 2015
This revised paperback and eBook edition published in 2017

Quote from *The Joy of Living: Unlocking the Secret & Science of Happiness*
by Yongey Rinpoche Mingyur and Eric Swanson; foreword by Daniel Goleman;
used with permission Penguin Random House.

ISBN 978-0-9968205-2-3
eBook ISBN 978-0-9968205-3-0

1. Self-Help / Self-Esteem
2. Personal Memoirs

Cover and design direction: Debbi Murzyn
Layout: Jo Marwick
Cover drawing: Pascale Chandler, Mielie, ink on paper

Say Yes Press

To the many special people who—often
unknowingly—have added an indelible mark
and given me reason to feel grateful.

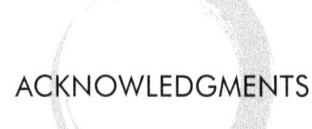

ACKNOWLEDGMENTS

Special thanks to:

Kathy Hrastar in Oakland, California for giving me a compelling deadline and being a star copy editor.

Rob Card in Canada, my former life coach, for helping me come up with a "life purpose" that gave me permission.

Anne Stevens in Durban, South Africa—with whom I've shared memorable culinary travel adventures in California and KwaZulu-Natal—for offering her superlative proofreading skills.

Debbi Murzyn in Pleasant Hill, California—design guru and friend—for her design direction and awesome cover.

Jo Marwick in Pietermaritzburg, South Africa—graphic designer and friend—for her creative formatting and layout ideas.

Alfons Hennig, my late dad, who taught me to appreciate good men and good food and who inadvertently gave me lots of stuff to work through.

Ryushin Paul Haller at San Francisco Zen Center for dharma inspiration and friendship. And to the many others who supported me at SFZC, including the late Hekizan Tom Girardot, always kind and pragmatic, who told me shortly after I moved in that "this is your home" and, impatiently, to "just hit it" when I was obsessing about getting my taiko bell rhythm "right."

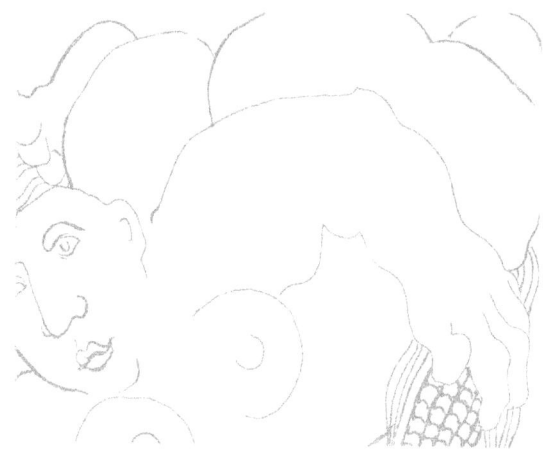

TABLE OF CONTENTS

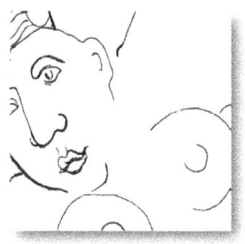

CHAPTER ONE

FOREPLAY

Paris with Helen starts as a nightmare. She wants to shop, shop, shop. I hate to shop but I want to be accommodating.

Thing is, I've been to Europe before, a couple of times. It's her first visit.

Plus, she's the cousin of my husband. The husband I'm meeting in London in a week's time. The husband under whose pillow I found a woman's nightie a week before he left, and I left, on our respective trips, him to the U.S. first, for work— something to do with computers—and me to Paris first, with Helen. A vacation from my job as a newspaper reporter in Durban, South Africa, and a break from being the mom of a cool daughter busy mastering the challenges of life in Grade 2.

Frumpy and sort of maiden-aunt homely the nightie was, I thought at the time, before I watched my mind run through: "Oh, he's having an affair.

"Good grief!

"New territory.

"How am I supposed to respond to this?

"Affair? Guidelines?

"Yes, you wanted to leave him.

"Yes, now you have grounds. You can blame him."

Oops! I watch my mind quickly hit delete; censor the tiny twinge of gloat and "gotcha, you bugger!" satisfaction.

"Don't rationalize," it tells me. "This is not the time to be calm and philosophical.

"Better to throw toys out of the pram. Have a tantrum."

Both of which I duly do.

So anyway, now I know this is going to be our one and only time in Europe, him and me together.

Which backstory I include to give a context to Helen, who I have traveled from South Africa with and who I'm spending my first five days with, staying on the outskirts of Paris, the last stop on the Métro line, with friends of her folks.

I like Helen. I like her parents. I might be planning to divorce her cousin. But I don't want to divorce the part of his family I like and who like me.

Hence my desire to be accommodating.

Which, then and now, is a tiresome tendency I can have.

When, finally, the time comes to head to Montmartre to have a bite, a glass of wine and listen to an accordion player, I am shopped out. I want to strangle Helen. Alternatively, jump off the Pont Neuf and drown myself.

So on Day Two, I say to Helen: "Let's split up and meet at 7 p.m."

Helen isn't keen. She's nervous to be alone in Paris. But sensing this is non-negotiable, she agrees.

Thus it is that we meet as planned, after dark, in the Pigalle.

〇

The Pigalle? The red light district? Two women in their twenties? Not hookers?

〇

OK. So Helen and I are in Paris back in the dark ages. That is, before South Africa's first democratic elections. It was an era when white supremacy in the form of apartheid ruled, Nelson Mandela was still in jail and many things were *verboten*, including pictures of him, any opposition to the then-government and, pertinent to this story, almost anything to do with sex.

Much happened covertly, as you might imagine.

A Miss Nude South Africa, for example—the jump-on-the-banned-wagon scheme of a used car salesman with friendly teeth (a smiley space between the front two). For a few short years it was an annual event in the tiny landlocked kingdom of Lesotho, the just-across-the-border destination for many South Africans drawn to porn, gambling and other "prohibitions."

And similar but more discreet, the strip show set up by an artist with a sense of humor and a penchant back then for sleaze and Jack Daniels. He organized it as a fund-raiser for the rugby club in the farming community spread around the rural hamlet of Winterton in KwaZulu-Natal.

Both the nudie gig and the strip show I got to attend incognito. By this I mean with my writer credentials purposefully not revealed. To the "body beautiful," because journalists had been banned after (what did they expect?) salacious stories in earlier years. And where, strange but true, I got invited to sit on the stage and be a judge.

I was invited by my roguish artist friend as a "stripper's assistant" to the rugby shebang, which event was secret to all but about 40 farmers who made their way to a hay barn somewhere in the middle of nowhere, plus the stripper who stripped, the hooker who hooked—both of whom were in on my subterfuge—the artist who set it all up but wasn't there, and me.

Secret until my story came out in an issue of Cosmopolitan mag.

But I digress again, once more in the interest of context.

◯

If something is forbidden, you want it. Right?

Whether you believe Bible stories are fiction, fable, or the truth, think of Eve and the apple. Forbidden fruit? What you resist, bring it on.

◯

Being from South Africa and curious if a bit green, Helen and I are drawn to explore the red light district. This includes seeing the Paris version of a blue movie, which we imagine will be, well, seriously blue.

And which we believe we've found when Helen elbows me and points to gilt-framed posters of erotically entwined nekkid bodies at a rather grand-looking cinema with an ornate façade, where you climb a pretty impressive flight of aged stone stairs and approach a wizened little French dame who looks like Jeanne Moreau gone wrong seated in a glassed-in ticket office.

The cinema's salubrious appearance is a welcome relief, the pair of us having, minutes before, escaped the clutches of a sweaty little man with a greasy comb-over who somehow (probably because we were polite and naive) propelled us into a claustrophobic confessional-cell-like booth off a narrow side street and gestured for us to peer through peepholes to where women, just like us but in the buff, were having sex with themselves and with each other on the floor, blatantly positioned to titillate those inclined (or prompted) to peek.

"I think he must want to offer us a job," I like to think I murmured to Helen.

I know we avoided eye contact with each other as we hot-footed it out of there, his lewd guffaws ringing in our ears.

⟳

"Ask if there are English subtitles," I tell Helen as we approach the movie cinema cashier.

A brief conversation ensues.

"She says no," Helen reports.

"Then ask her if there's another movie later with English subtitles," I say.

Helen turns back toward the glass partition and another exchange takes place.

"She says no. No subtitles. No English. She seems to be saying there's no need," Helen reports back.

Her confusion matches my indignation.

"That's ridiculous," I pronounce, glaring at Ms. Moreau in her glassed-in box. "Let's go find a better movie house."

I don't know what I mean by "better" given that this one looks pretty plush. And after walking a couple of blocks, on tired feet in boots with heels that we've been walking in all day, we head back.

Was it my imagination or was Ms. Moreau smirking when she handed Helen our tickets?

Think of it from her perspective. Profound discussion between two young women, a blonde and a brunette, who definitely aren't French, although one has a pidgin version and probably fancies herself as a linguist. Her only women customers all day if not all week or perhaps all year. Both very earnest and preoccupied with—English subtitles.

We go in. I look around, peering into darkness illuminated by the screen. I note that we are the only women in the place. The sprinkling of men—were they really all wearing dark raincoats and looking desperate, as my memory suggests?

Some credits roll and the film begins.

And what do we have?

Naked women in a kitchen.

Not barefoot and pregnant, but barefoot and preparing food.

Bowls are out.

And blenders. And slicers.

Action.
Take One: Bananas.

Take Two: English cucumbers.

Take Three: I never did find carrots sexy so let's forget about them and the rest of the ingredients.

Turns out we have walked in on a porn movie. One where a bunch of women are about to have sex.

Wait.

Now they're having sex.

And not just sex, but what looks like incredibly satisfying sex.

With vegetables.

And when they're done with the veggies, the women slice them and dice them and toss up a salad.

At which point naked men arrive and the men and women eat the salad.

Then at some point the women have sex with the men.

But you know, I don't remember the men. Or the sex with the men. Or anything about the film that followed.

I have, on the other hand, never managed to look at a banana or any form of cucumber to this day without thinking: "Hmm, is anyone else seeing just a banana? Simply a cuke?"

When we left that movie house in Paris, Ms. Moreau's cackling followed us down the street. I wonder why.

◯

Sex and food. Food and sex. Embracing, like reluctant Siamese twins. For many women food and sex have become the intimate coupling. And not just women. Seems more men describe culinary experiences as "orgasmic."

Nothing orgasmic about binge eating, though. And nothing even vaguely sexy about visits from the black dog. Or by being gutted randomly, often, and even in intimate settings and benign social situations by an extreme form of "stage fright," although social anxiety disorder is likely the appropriate label. Dark places, interdependent and interconnected.

I reckon the seed that grew into a solution—and liberation—was planted the night Helen and I vegged out in Paris.

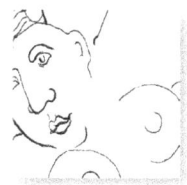

CHAPTER TWO

GROPING IN THE DARK

Fast-forward 15 years from Paris, France to a waterbed in
Pocatello, Idaho. My very first waterbed experience. Did I
see it in some movie? Or maybe the idea came from a book.
A motel room bedecked with spangled hearts and flaming
fuchsias. Click a switch for soft music and pulp porn. In pride
of place is a great big waterbed that, when you put quarters in
a slot, begins to jiggle and gyrate.

Not surprisingly, this being potato country, my Pocatello
waterbed has about as much in common with the waterbed
of my fantasy as a limp leftover Lay's does with a plump
barbecue-baked Idaho russet smothered with crispy bacon bits
and dolloped with salty butter and the freshest sour cream. Not
a panting petunia or a breathless begonia in sight.

For a start, it is in the basement of a Mormon family's
house. Then, it's a single bed dispassionately clad in brown.

Its owner, a young man I have not met, is somewhere in the
world doing his Mormon mission.

I am, at the time, new to the United States and on a
journey via Greyhound discovering small-town America. The

bulk of my "stuff"—what I brought from South Africa, plus a laptop purchased from Radio Shack upon arrival—is at the San Francisco Zen Center.

When I landed at SFO five months previously with a one-year return ticket and a 10-year visitor's visa, I had the SFZC address scribbled in a notebook but no idea I'd become a Zen student and live and practice there for going on four years.

The bus adventure wasn't on my agenda either.

But here I was in Pocatello, a place I'd never heard of before my friend June, a long-lapsed Mormon I'd worked with on a newspaper in Durban, arranged for me to stay overnight with her true-blue Mormon sister's family.

Being alone in his waterbed meant I could toss and turn and bounce and roll and enjoy the pulsations of my animated sleeper, and eventually h-e-a-v-e myself onto my stomach. Which is when it happened.

Was it the novelty?

Possibly.

The movement?

Probably.

Anyway, as I landed a-quiver on my belly, an unexpected sexual tingling informed me that I was feeling turned on.

What followed was a sequence of woolly and what at first seemed disconnected observations, which then began to slot into place like a jigsaw.

Feeling sexy made me think of sex. This reminded me that I was alone and, in my aloneness, as celibate as a Mother Superior. Apt, given that I'd been plunked, at age seven, into a boarding school with nuns. And given that before leaving for the United States, in the interests of self-preservation and having had one too many libido-driven hellish relationship, I had pledged myself to a year of celibacy.

I reckon it's safe to assume we've all heard the old "Life begins at 40" maxim? Well there I was, on the cusp.

And how did I feel at age 40?

Like I'd been there, done that—and now what? Career, motherhood, marriage, divorce, relationships; a protracted stint in therapy trying to fathom the meaning of it all. I could honestly say my life had been full, rich, intense, angst-riddled, funny and varied.

Enough already. Couldn't we, it and me, curl up in a fetal under the duvet and stay there? D'you know what I mean?

But for better or worse, I was in pretty good nick physically and mentally, all things considered. And life? It has this habit of waking up with us each morning—like in *Groundhog Day*—for who knows how long?

It seemed the time had come to take the plunge; give my life a helping hand.

I'd thought of going to London where a guy friend had said, "Come stay—as long as you like."

When I mention this to a girlfriend who's recently moved to San Francisco for a man, she says why not come instead to California? She has an office space I can use as a base. "His ex was a writer. She left him for a woman," she tells me, adding that she, my friend, is meant to fill the work gap as well as the other gaps.

"And I can't write but you can," she says, which is true. "Come quick as you can," she urges in calls and faxes, telling me she's miserable and could use a friend. Her new bloke's field is diversity training, which will mean a shift in direction for me and I am keen on a new career challenge.

So it is that within six weeks of never having considered visiting the U.S., I leave Durban and travel halfway around the world. A couple of South African editors have said they'll buy any decent stories I send back. My daughter, three years out of high school and at university, has said she will be happy to have a journalist friend of mine plus a post-grad student gleaned via a newspaper ad move in to share our apartment and help with the rent. Her dad lives an hour away; her gran a lot closer.

I get myself a one-year return ticket and decide to call what I'm doing a sabbatical.

Somewhere this will switch for a time to midlife crisis.

Why? No special reason. It would just seem I was in the right place at the right time to have one of these. And we do like labels, don't we?

I travel via London. The night before I am due to fly on, my San Francisco buddy calls me. She says her new mate has been pressing her to tell me not to come.

Too late. No going back now. And as it turns out fate has more interesting things in store than the chilly basement studio and frosty reception that is waiting.

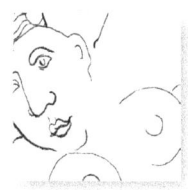

CHAPTER THREE

HONEY DON'T

"If you don't run, run, run, you're going to commit suicide."
I'm at the Buddhist Retreat Center—the BRC—in rural Ixopo, South Africa. If you ever chanced upon Alan Paton's classic novel, *Cry, the Beloved Country*, you might recognize the name Ixopo. It's the setting for the book's opener.

> "There is a lovely road that runs from Ixopo into the hills.
> These hills are grass-covered and rolling, and they are lovely
> beyond any singing of it. The road climbs seven miles into
> them, to Carisbrooke; and from there, if there is no mist, you
> look down on one of the fairest valleys of Africa."
> —Alan Paton, Cry, the Beloved Country.

I'm sitting by the stupa overlooking a sweeping KwaZulu-Natal valley, with its distant patchwork of modest mud and thatch family compounds clinging to erosion-ravaged hillsides, when the words of warning shock me out of what I could have sworn was safe invisibility.

A bee, the motherfucker, has stung my right hand. The affected part has swollen to the size of a tennis ball. The suicide remark comes just as I'm pondering one of life's mysteries: bee is dead and I am in pain. Who is better off?

Because it is painful. But the physical pain is not the issue.

What is, is the embarrassment. The fear of attention. The anxiety at the prospect of someone seeing and making a fuss. If I'm allergic, better to just die. Quickly.

None of this is morbid. On the contrary, it's familiar territory.

But yes, I am also depressed, this time round for some weeks.

I once told my mother I was feeling, not depressed—because that is not an easy word to use—but very down. "How can you say that when you're so lucky," she countered. "Count your blessings."

And indeed, I don't tell people when I'm depressed. I feel embarrassed to say it. There are so many people around who have real problems. Like those in that valley you look down on from the BRC. The valley from which an abstruse soundtrack drifts into the meditation hall on Sunday mornings: of people pounding on cowhide drums. I am very aware of real suffering, of poverty, of the "There but for the grace of God" realities of this world.

Besides, who wants to be with people who wear their dejection like a shroud? Who wants to really know when they say "How are you?" that you're depressed?

◯

I will come to learn a lot about depression. I will learn, but only way in the future, to identify the brooding pattern that can dip one into the dark pit. I will learn this while researching Zen, mindfulness and depression to write a grant proposal many years later for a San Francisco Zen Center—SFZC—abbot.

By then I will also understand that the black dog is a hovering presence. And that life isn't worth living if I let myself be nudged over the edge and onto what I will come to think of as the slippery slide.

*

At the time of the bee sting, the depression is the worst it's been in ages. The needle is stuck in the same groove of an old vinyl record. It's playing the same furrow over and over again, digging in deeper and deeper. Dig deep enough for long enough, at some point what you're focused on is likely to become a self-fulfilling prophecy.

Tossie, the therapist leading the creativity retreat I'm at the BRC to do, has no idea how her words resonate when she spots me sitting alone, notices my hand and reads beyond my hand, beyond my public smiley-face, to something I had thought I was successfully hiding.

Having said that, being "seen" gives me an unaccountable sense of relief. Sort of like a perfectly positioned strike with the *kyosaku* on your aching back when you're meditating in the zendo. It, like, reverbs through the muscle paths and wakes up all of you.

At the time, this *kyosaku* wake-up experience is also in my future.

*

The next day I pick up a book in the BRC library by a Korean Zen teacher. He talks about depression.

He says to think of it as someone you know—an acquaintance—who knocks at the door. You invite him in. You engage. You listen. You share a cuppa.

Then you say cheers and see him out.

You don't invite him to move in and stay.

Somewhere else, I read the groove in the vinyl record reference.

You hear a couple of things like this, they make sense. I started to force a shift out of the groove. A year later, when I bought my ticket to ride, I didn't think of it as running, but looking back, it was. I ran, ran, ran away—to San Francisco.

⟲

Back on that waterbed in Pocatello, my thoughts switched unexpectedly to food, which caused me to think of my ballooning midriff and my most recent bout of bingeing.

I knew it was comfort eating, but being aware didn't help.

"I need comfort and this is comforting," I'd been telling myself when, as a newbie in an unfamiliar country with things not going as planned, the chocolate bars, second helpings, midnight snacks—and more novelty American junk food from more fast-food outlets than a souped-up ADHD brain on a sugar high could conceive of—vanished into my mouth.

Lying there, the notion of comfort made me think of nurturing.

A big bear hug. A gentle caress.

The pleasure of this image made me think again of food.

Specifically, of the kitchen fridge humming with full-bellied contentment in a room above my waterbed.

Could I, a guest in a virtual stranger's home, justify raiding it? Could I justify raiding it after the substantial three-course meal we'd had for dinner? Not bloody likely.

◯

Food and sex. In the absence of more food, I returned to feeling sexual and into my mind, from my grad school days, jumped Maslow. Namely, psychologist Abraham Maslow. His "hierarchy of needs," required reading years back when I was a psych student, popped from some obtuse storage space in my brain. Maslow's hierarchy that, in effect, places a person's physiological needs—for oxygen, water, food, sex and sleep— at the base of a pyramid from where they dominate and dictate behavior until met.

At which stage higher needs—for safety, affection, esteem and so forth—arise and call the tune.

At the pinnacle he placed self-actualization, which at first encounter I wanted because clearly, this was the cherry on the top.

But back to food and sex that night; those primal drives integral to species survival. Thinking of them side by side got me wondering just how equal they were.

How equal were they supposed to be?

And what happened when they went out of kilter and one subsumed the other?

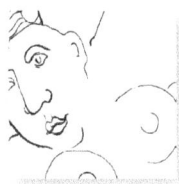

CHAPTER FOUR

TURNED ON AND TUNED IN

It's New Year's Eve at San Francisco's War Memorial Opera House where, in 1945, representatives of 50 nations assembled to sign the Charter of the United Nations. Tonight the "Green Room" is the venue of the Gay, Lesbian, Bisexual and Transgender Alcoholics Anonymous Ball. I am none of these but it's my first New Year's Eve in California. I am living at SFZC. And when a woman from Minnesota, a Zen student who has come to live in the building for a while, says "You wanna go dance? It's close enough to walk," it seems profoundly San Francisco perfect.

As I try to get my body in tune with the music, I feel awkward and self-conscious, not knowing how to be on the dance floor with my new friend, feeling an impostor in this room, wishing I had natural rhythm. Then I remind myself of where I am, which makes me smile, and look around and become aware that nobody is even vaguely interested in me, including my friend who is contorting in her own public-private space. I tell myself to cut the crap and just breathe.

And all of a sudden I slip into a different place. There is acute awareness that I am on the other side of the world, about equidistant either way, in fact, from where I've come. I start to feel the music in my body. My body seems to grow bigger, stronger. And I become aware of a lightness of being infused with energy and power.

This feeling has a voice.

The voice is saying: "Don't fuck with me, world."

Odd. Or is it?

○

Go back one year. It's New Year's morning. I am climbing Table Mountain in Cape Town, angry at my prick of a boyfriend who's been smoking pot and stoned out of his tree for three days straight. Why did he fly to Durban so we could drive the 1,050 miles together to his place in Cape Town for New Year if he was planning to not "be there?"

It made for yet another gloomy New Year's Eve. One which, when I left my ill humor for rare moments of detached observation, I saw could have been magical with different companions. Or with the same ones, were I also a dopehead.

Or if I could have found my sense of humor, lightened up, or—easy to be wise with hindsight—got out of my funk, found other people to talk to or things to feel grateful for. Our table, after all, was right on the water's edge at a Cape Town waterfront restaurant. Sailboats with revelers. Fireworks at midnight. Balmy weather. Abundant bubbly. Probably there was moonshine. Maybe even stardust. And people dressed to party.

Beautiful people—a TV ad setting.

But, oh, blah is me.

Then the next morning, fueled with pissed-off energy, climbing, scrambling, strong, exhilarated, muscles, strength, sweat. Remembering that one year before, I had also been in Cape Town for New Year. And at Table Mountain.

The present boyfriend, then, was not yet a blip on the radar.

The previous boyfriend and I had dragged on—and on— probably five years beyond implosion. It was finally over and I was still pulling myself out of the rubble.

⟁

That time round, I didn't hike up Table Mountain. We reached the peak by cable car. I'd driven to Cape Town with my daughter. Same drive; different companion. Some new friends she'd made suggested going to the top of Table Mountain to drink wine and watch the sunset.

But it was wasted on me. I sat away from my daughter's group, grateful they'd twisted my arm to go with them, but off on my own rock. Not drinking wine because, given that I was older, I should have bought the wine and should not drink theirs. No?

And entertaining myself by playing out fantasies that involved diving over the edge and falling down, down, down to oblivion.

But convention ruled, not drama, and I took the cable car.

⟁

Fast-forward one year. Same mountain. Different space.

The boyfriend and his buddies from last night, my companions on the cliff face this morning, become incidental as I climb, climb, up and up, on this first morning of this New Year. Myself on this mountain in the sunshine. I feel on the verge—of a new life.

⟲

Six weeks after that mountain metamorphosis I consult with my daughter about leaving home for a year.

Not her. Me.

In practical terms there's "empty nest" to confront. Single mom. Enmeshment. You know you need to push them out; empower them. Easier said than done if the status quo doesn't change.

Then came my first job layoff.

Work and motherhood. My focus, my purpose, my two long-time escape routes—from "me." Both had folded in on themselves.

Four weeks after our confab, the two seemingly fitting roommates are ready to move in. The kitchen is plastered with signs: "Have you hugged and fed your Passion today?" Passion being our chocolate-brown toy poodle. Everything possible to arrange has been arranged, farewell drinks drunk, goodbye dinners savored. And I bid my temporary farewell.

On April Fool's Day I touch down in San Francisco knowing little about the place besides some song lyrics, that it has steep streets, that it has an island prison same as Cape Town, and that there had been a lot of hippies here in the days we wore flowers in our hair in Durban.

Oh, and in addition to the address of SFZC, jotted down on my final visit to the Buddhist Retreat Center before I leave, I have in my suitcase a book called *Zen Mind, Beginners Mind* by Shunryu Suzuki.

"The purpose of Buddhism is not to study Buddhism, but to study ourselves."—Zen Mind, Beginner's Mind by Shunryu Suzuki, founder of the San Francisco Zen Center.

If anyone had suggested, the New Year's morning I hiked up Table Mountain, that within a year I would have traveled a chunk of the United States when I had always said I would never go there as it was too big to know where to start, and that I'd be living in a Zen temple, I would have thought they'd been doing some magical version of mushrooms.

Before I leave, the single most common sound bite I hear when I mention San Francisco—other than the "take condoms" litany, which seems to be the fate of the single woman—is "bald heads." I am too busy tying up loose ends to give the city a face but it quickly develops features as friends and acquaintances speak of Victorian facades, summer fog, sheer streets, cable cars—and bald heads.

"It's the AIDS capital of the world," several people tell me, forgetting that we're living in Africa where HIV/AIDS has wiped out entire villages.

If I'd believed my ears, I might have imagined a sea of stubbly orbs floating disconnected through the streets of San Francisco.

As it turns out, I meet a lot of bald heads and I meet a lot of people with HIV. Most of those with HIV have hair.

Most of those with bald heads fall into one of two categories. Either they are modern primitives and punks making fashion statements. Or they are men and women Zen Buddhist monks. Most of the bald heads I become intimate with belong to fellow monks.

○

San Francisco Zen Center came into being in 1962, three years after Shunryu Suzuki, a Japanese Zen Buddhist priest, arrived to serve the city's Japanese community and let it be known that anyone interested could come sit zazen (Zen meditation) with him. Destined to write *Zen Mind, Beginner's Mind*, for many years the best-selling book on Zen in English—and the book that, by chance, I popped into my suitcase to take to San Francisco—the story goes that he was soon joined by a growing band of barefoot and hairy hippie-type men and women. Among them were poets, artists, writers, musicians and varied drop-outs. At some stage they grew into a stable community.

In 1967, wanting a monastery, they raised funds with the help of a "Zenefit," a rock concert featuring a line-up of supporters including Big Brother and the Holding Company and Jefferson Airplane. They bought Tassajara, a hot springs resort in California's Carmel Valley, which became the first residential Zen-training center in the West, popularly known for its innovative vegetarian kitchen.

In 1969, in need of a city residential practice center, they bought 300 Page Street and called it Beginner's Mind Temple. This became home to SFZC's City Center and, going on three decades later, to me. A capacious red brick place that breathes tranquility in sometimes turbulent surrounds, the building was designed at the turn of the last century by California architect Julia Morgan, more famous for her work on Hearst Castle, as a residential home for young Jewish girls.

There it was, in the heart of the city that in its hippy-dippy make-love-and-not-war phase, one-time drug culture exponent Timothy Leary tagged the most progressive, liberal, open-minded, experimental, future-oriented city in the world and the probe of the human species into the 21st century. If you were a young Jewish girl in San Francisco in 1969, probably the last thing you wanted was a cloistered residence.

Which is why the place was up for sale.

○

Looking back to the early Nineties when I moved in, "multiple" seems apt when putting personality to Zen Center's environs.

The four-way stop outside the front door was a round-the-clock pick-up point for prostitutes. One block up was a "project," as the city called its low-cost housing hotbeds of crime and drugs. Robert Pirsig, in his 1970s' classic *Zen and the Art of Motorcycle Maintenance*, relates a journey with his young son Chris. It was outside this project some years later that the selfsame Chris, staying at SFZC at the time, was fatally stabbed.

On a more auspicious note, a gracious Victorian nearby housed—still does—the Zen Hospice Project, which offered hospice training and a chance to volunteer. A walk from SFZC to "the Castro," often referred to as the gay capital of the world, will take you maybe 20 minutes. A fast 10 minutes in another direction and you're at Civic Center, home to a cluster of landmark locations, including City Hall, the symphony hall, opera house, main library and Asian Art Museum. It's a 20-minute speedy stroll to the heart of the Haight-Ashbury, which peaked in 1966 as the flower power, free love, drug and hippie center of the world. A brisk urban hike of less than an hour and you're in bohemian North Beach, home of City Lights, the still-going-strong bookstore founded by poet Lawrence Ferlinghetti (with college prof Peter D. Martin) that became the hub of the Beat generation in the Fifties and a hangout for Allen Ginsberg (*Howl and Other Poems*) and Jack Kerouac (*On the Road* and *The Dharma Bums*) in their heyday.

You live in the city, you learn to walk it well. That is, not as the crow flies.

It may be notorious for its steep streets and you can climb them if you dare. But as with many things in life, there are alternative highways, byways and routes from A to B that might seem counter-intuitive—but make the journey sweeter.

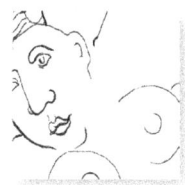

CHAPTER FIVE

ALL FIRED UP

I first rang the doorbell at 300 Page Street about three weeks after getting to San Francisco and right off became a regular at the Saturday program of zazen, lecture and lunch. A couple of months later I asked if I might move in. They said OK. And so I did, with suitcases and a sleeping bag bought from a camping store on Market Street, as a guest student.

Most rooms were singles, furnished with a futon. Rent included your meals. And life was an ongoing lesson in impermanence as scatterlings, not only from Africa but also from Australia, Asia, Great Britain, Canada and all over America, moved in and moved on.

To be one of this united nations of guest students meant you paid less rent than did residents—my subsequent status except for when, as a "scholarship" student, I paid in time and kind, sewing more zafus and zabutans than there were butts to sit on them.

In all these capacities, you got to rise daily at 4:50 a.m. for morning zazen. You undertook to attend a prescribed number of lectures each week, partake in a monthly all-day zazen program, and if your tenure happened to coincide, join occasional meditation marathons called sesshins that lasted all week.

As with any community where everyone shares the load, you got included in the weekly roster of tasks which, this being a temple, might include bell-ringing, drum-pounding and doing things with incense. They sound benign enough but time and again the prospect of doing them—doing them wrong—would send me into a flat spin and give rise to hot sweats, angst-filled nights and palpitations.

In addition, in this community where the most common complaint was sleep deprivation, as a guest student you got to do chores: specifically, the general scrubbing, cleaning, cooking and polishing of housework.

If you'd quizzed me before I left Durban on where I'd find myself living in the U.S., a temple would never have made it onto the list. Twelve years of education at a convent girls' school with nuns had cured me of "religion." And I think of myself as more carnal than spiritual.

On the other hand, I'd long been interested in meditation—having noted that people who meditated were focused, often out-the-box, and grounded by some seemingly secret inner strength. From my teen years I'd been pondering the meaning of life (neither a therapist nor Monty Python had shed light). I think part of the draw of meditation was a sense that any meaning to be found was "in here;" not "out there."

And I would discover from listening to the weekly student talks (new arrivals were asked to share "How I got to Zen

Center") that not only questioning people, but also people searching for freedom from painful angst, gravitate to Zen.

I had come to understand that Buddhism sat comfortably with no religion or any religion and attracted more than its fair share of retired Catholics like myself, and Jews. I knew I could embrace it without feigning piousness.

And Zen and meditation? I came to understand that to all intents and purposes, they were one and the same.

I'd been at Zen Center no more than a couple of weeks when Satish Kumar came to stay. In the 60s, Kumar undertook an 8,000-mile peace pilgrimage. Carrying no money and depending on the kindness of strangers he walked from Gandhi's tomb in his native India to Moscow, Paris, London and Washington, D.C. (crossing the Atlantic on the Queen Mary), delivering packets of "peace tea" to the leaders of these nuclear powers.

Kumar, co-founder and director of England's eco-spiritual Schumacher College, mentioned in a talk that it was common for Indian men of around age 40 with grown-up kids to leave home on spiritual quests.

What was I doing? I asked myself many times in those early days, trying to justify cleaning loos and polishing clean windows at Zen Center in place of pursuing my career. Funny how uncomfortable we feel without handy tags. I liked the idea of what these Indian guys were doing. I tried it on for size.

But if truth be told, it sounded like a male cop-out. And as I've said before, I didn't class myself as spiritual.

So what could I call my adventure?

Finding a new vocation?

I recall testing this one as I diligently peeled yet another broccoli stem with a small paring knife and tried to appreciate all that had gone into creating this broccoli stem and getting it to the chopping board. When you cooked and cleaned at Zen Center, you were urged to "just do" what you were doing, which meant doing it in silence and becoming one with what you were doing.

I was surprised to find that when all I did was cook or clean, it became intensely satisfying work. I pondered the idea of adding a practical skill to my resume: "American-trained domestic worker with Zen-infused Japanese skills."

Then at some point, I gave up on the labels. Might as well accept that at this time and in this space, the inner journey had become more compelling than the outer one.

◯

Meanwhile, living in a temple quickly became commonplace, give or take a few dozen prostrations each week and some unusual ceremonies like the one at Halloween when the Zen honchos blew horns and conches, banged a weird assortment of instruments, waved horsehair fly whisks, and lured the ghosts of the dead with bowls of fruit and sweets.

◯

I especially liked the Zen New Year ritual. After sitting cross-legged facing the wall in the run-up to midnight, attending to the breath (like Cinderella, my Minnesota friend and I made it back from the ball in time) and hearing from this quiet place the city rise in a crescendo of blaring hooters and boom-boxes, everybody moved to Zen Center's enclosed courtyard that opens to the stars. Here, someone lit a lively fire in a giant kitchen wok. To hell with New Year's resolutions you're never going to keep. Rather, write down your bad habits from the old year and burn 'em. List the bad relationships and roast 'em. Say good riddance, then start the year afresh.

And living at Zen Center? I learned that it takes all types to make a temple. From the committed contemplatives to the earnest 40-something computer-whizz rock guitarist father-of-two who went out and got Buddha eyes tattooed on the back of his shaven head. From the conservative jocks to the young, gay, aspiring financier who told me that his scrotum ring was "for aesthetic appeal," his nipple rings "for added sensation" and his tongue stud "to give my lovers pleasure."

I experienced first-hand the truism that you need to live with people to know them. And living together is a great leveler.

At first I was surprised when talk at the monthly house meeting dwelled for 40 minutes on the kitchen roaches followed by 20 minutes on why we couldn't have a microwave: because someone would break it. (We got one and somebody broke it.)

Soon I grew accustomed to being surprised. And when my daughter, back in South Africa, spread her wings wider than expected and went off on a journey of her own, the temple became my home for two years, and then another year—and into a fourth; the community my extended family.

⟳

My friends, meanwhile, got used to the idea that I was there. No longer did I get the solicitous "Are you sure you're OK?" when I gave them my address.

Some optimistic males talked of moving in when they heard that actress Uma Thurman's dad, Robert, was a professor of Tibetan Buddhism and sometimes came to speak. A woman friend wanted to cross the ocean and take vows when she heard actor Peter Coyote had been known to drop by.

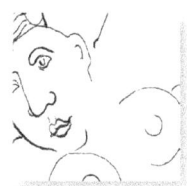

CHAPTER SIX

FATAL DISTRACTION

D o I want food—or do I want sex?
       This pops from somewhere unconscious or
subconscious and becomes my mantra after my night on the
waterbed in Pocatello.

The thing is, by then I have been going "on diet" for as
long as I can remember. Diet not in the old-fashioned sense:
what my version of Webster's describes as "Food and drink
considered in terms of its qualities, composition, and its effects
on health as in 'Milk is a wholesome article of diet.'"

I'm talking diet, the four-letter word. Namely:

D as in Deprive yourself and you are Depraved if you don't;

I as in Isolate and Insulate yourself with food;

E as in if it tastes good it must be Evil to Eat it; and

T as in Torture yourself to Thinness.

Diet milkshakes, slimming clubs, massage machines, diet
pills, laser slimming, kelp, fiber tabs, fasting, purging, calorie
counting, laxatives, no-fat, high-fat, diet trends from paleo
and protein to meat-focused, vegan and raw. From grapes

to grapefruit and from the 10-minute diet dash to the 10-month diet marathon. Name it and I'd tried it.

I'd read books, counted calories and tried products, from suppressants to saccharin and stevia. I'd bumped and ground my way through exercise classes done not for the pleasure of the doing, but with the specific focus on "results."

I'd found it easy to go on a diet. So easy, I was inclined to start a new one every Monday (and give it up on Tuesday). Call me the Diet Queen. No joke. I'd lost so many pounds on so many diets over so many years—more in total than my body weight (I once did a calculation)—I should have been a shadow of myself. Yet I was as dissatisfied with my shape as ever.

And when I was on a diet? I could recall, a dozen years later, the precise number of fish eggs on a sandwich that I clenched my jaws and declined at a cocktail party while toiling through a week-long regime that restricted me to apples.

The problem was that "diet," as in the four-letter word, was never far from my agenda. I was either "on diet" or "off diet." This was more complicated than it sounds because "on diet" invariably meant waiting to go "off diet," while "off diet" meant preparing to go "on diet." Adding to this, "on diet" had the connotation of being good, as in disciplined, while "off diet" was bad, as in decadent.

But I *liked* decadent. I didn't like disciplined. And "on diet" invariably felt like punishment and deprivation while "off diet" had many moments of pleasure—but caused pain.

○

Meanwhile, in a world that had been eluding me, the "no diet" route beckoned. Eat precisely what you feel like when you're hungry and stop as soon as your tummy is comfortably full. This, I was convinced, was really the way to go.

I'd tried it, many times, but to no avail. The thing is—or more aptly was—that after years of nymphonoshing, blocking my feelings with food, hiding my shyness and insecurities behind food (eat to bloat at a dinner party, the physical discomfort consumes the social discomfort), eating for just about any reason other than hunger, I'd lost touch with my body's needs and rhythms.

⟳

Do I want food—or do I want sex?

The mantra arrived, as I say, unsolicited. In the context of my Pocatello "awakening," which is what it had felt like, it made sense. And I was ready.

My next Greyhound bus stop after Pocatello was Salt Lake City. I got off right in the downtown area. It was around lunchtime.

What do you do when you're alone in a city you don't know with time on your hands?

If food is your focus, hungry or not hungry, your default is to go eat.

"Do I want food or do I want sex?" I asked myself. The question put me in my body, which I had to tune into, to get an answer.

The answer was loud and clear.

Sex.

This gave me a yardstick.

So, I wasn't really and truly hungry.

But habit or whatever, I still wanted to eat something.

I went into a diner near the temple. I scanned the menu. I examined the dessert trolley and noticed a luscious airy-looking cake piled with fresh whipped cream and strawberries. I looked back at the lunch menu.

Logic and "rules" told me that I should have some "real food" and then the strawberry cake for dessert.

My body told me it wasn't hungry for all that. What I really felt like when I thought about chewing, eating and digesting the different options, was the cake.

So that's what I ordered.

I felt a little naughty as I savored it; relished it. The strawberries were sweet and succulent. The cream was thick with a hint of sweetness and melt-in-the-mouth delish. The sponge was mouthwatering and light.

I felt I had made a tiny breakthrough.

◯

Do I want food—or do I want sex?

I knew long before I got to the U.S. that diets don't work. As I say, I'd been there, done that, so many times, over so many years.

"Eat exactly what you want when you are hungry and stop when you have had enough."

This made total sense to me.

But as often as I'd tried to rely on my stomach-hunger cues, I'd failed.

Babies cry when they're hungry and stop eating, if we let them, when they've had enough. I was once a baby. It made sense those innate prompts were still there—somewhere.

The first "don't diet" book I read was British psychotherapist Susie Orbach's *Fat is a Feminist Issue* w-a-y before she worked with the late Princess Diana when Diana was alive and not too well, being married to Charles, and battling an eating disorder. Orbach's drift, as I related to it, was to stop treating certain foods as taboo and to wait for your stomach to signal when you were hungry and what you were hungry for.

You were to stop eating not when the plate had been scraped clean—(albeit for the starving children in Ethiopia)—but when your stomach told you it was comfortably satisfied.

I was working in the newsroom of a daily newspaper in South Africa when I first read Orbach's book and decided that I would focus deep attention on my belly: I'd only eat when it told me to—and stop when it informed me I had fed it an elegant sufficiency (in contrast to starving it, or gobbling down a piggish amount).

But there was one indigestible problem.

I would wait and wait—and my hunger failed to ping at me, let alone exert a resounding pang.

At lunchtime when friends said "let's go to the canteen," I couldn't. Neither could I tell them why I couldn't. That I was waiting for my stomach to speak to me. The idea of such a confession was absurd.

And it was beyond my scope to imagine going to the canteen and not eating.

The fourth day this happened and I saw them disappearing down the stairs, I followed—and devoured something diabolical like curry gravy over a steak and kidney pie and fat greasy fries.

Perhaps I was too impatient. Maybe I lacked persistence and should have waited. What? Several months?

Whatever, I found my stomach cues impossible to detect. I knew absolutely that Orbach was right. I knew I had to stop dieting. I knew I had to listen to my body.

It was just going to take a long time to find a way to tune into my body that worked for me.

⟳

Do I want food—or do I want sex?

After some time, I found that with this shorthand, I was able to create a shift in focus from my former compulsions.

Is it because eating is physical and sex is physical? Eating is nurturing and sex is nurturing. Eating is for pleasure and sex is for pleasure (in both cases when we give ourselves the permission). Eating is company and sex is company. Eating is earthy and sex is earthy. Eating is now and feeling sexual is now. Both eating and sex are tangible realities.

When I turned on and tuned into myself as a sexual and sensual being—not in terms of a real or fantasy man, present or absent, but just experiencing myself as a sexual and sensual being in relationship with my world—I found I became more in-the-moment present; less into my head, habits and compulsions. Along with this, I became aware that I was beginning to feel my body's rhythms.

Which gets to the heart of the matter.

○

Because, let's face it, no matter how much we feed either of our hungry mouths, oral or vaginal, if we are feeding the deprivations of an inner child, we'll never feel satisfied and fulfilled. If our hunger is in fact for comfort, for connection, for love, for escape, for reward, we'll keep craving more. If we're eating to run away from uncomfortable feelings like shyness, isolation, bleakness or one of any number of personal inadequacies, we're still going to be hungry when we're done.

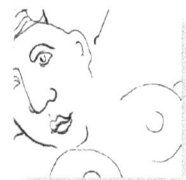

CHAPTER SEVEN

SPLICED

"**O**ral and vaginal—the two hungry mouths."

Thank you for that, Helen.

Not the Paris Helen. This time it's therapist Helen.

Zip forward a couple of dozen years from the Pigalle and a couple of months from Pocatello.

I am back at SFZC developing high blood pressure (seriously!) t-r-y-i-n-g (far too hard) to meditate "properly." More about that later.

And committed to being celibate for a year.

The celibacy has nothing to do with living in a temple, aka a monastery, which means we are all, essentially, monks. There is a Zen precept that suggests you "not misuse sexuality," but, rather, "cultivate and encourage open and honest relationships." The Zen precepts are like Zen commandments, except they're not rules. There's no fire-and-brimstone suffer-in-hell prospect in an afterlife if you break them. Taking them on is optional and effected through a ceremony called *jukai* in which you commit to the intention of living by them and are given a Japanese name by your practice leader, basically your Zen mentor: typically a priest.

So, while sexuality is addressed, celibacy is not a Zen requirement.

On the contrary, given several dalliances one couldn't help but notice when living in sort of a goldfish bowl, no matter how discreet you tried to be or they tried to be, which is probably a feature of living communally anywhere. And how many hours a day, I wonder, did the lovably mordant not-so-young gay monk—who ran the sewing room where I stitched and stuffed zafus and zabutans day after day for some months—spend gently to wildly obsessing about the stodgily hunky young straight monk who worked in the kitchen? So many sighs, so many utterances of adoration, so many comments about hot biceps (really?) and kissable lips (what?) that finally, at some point, the kitchen guy, who I'm pretty friendly with and who has never been anything but blobby, transforms into a sex object for me, too, after a night of tequila shots in the Mission.

But that is in the future, after my year's celibacy commitment has runneth over. So enough about that.

Although the scenario did make me wonder how many affairs are sparked by someone waxing lyrical to a best friend about their significant other's perceived attributes.

Be that as it may, the celibacy proves to be an unexpected life-changer. Only child. All-girls school. Nuns who warned you about boys. A dad who worked hard, spoke little. A mom who didn't like him, poor man. Passive-aggressive comes from women too. And some women use and abuse men, same as the other way round. Maybe not as often physically, but emotionally, certainly. (Sorry, sisters, if you disagree.)

Far easier to jump into bed with boys than talk to them. Can I say that? Embarrassing to divulge one's shadow side and vulnerabilities.

But I have learned that whenever I share a secret shame, likely a product of deep-rooted Catholic guilt, there are others who claim it is their secret shame as well. If I admit to a major shortcoming or confess a failing, there are others who express relief that it's not just them, which I also feel when it happens in reverse.

And those who are going to judge will judge, come what may.

Being celibate, I get more comfortable with myself, and with men, and in the company of men. And it gets me beyond my default mode of seeing attractive men as sex objects and clamming up, running away or rolling over. And beyond seeing "boyfriend men" as my mom saw my dad, which was as an adversary.

⟲

I return to San Francisco in a state of private excitement. Private because while my new eating practices make sense experientially, articulating things verbally is my block. Writing works because it is simply about rooting out what I am sensing or feeling or experiencing for my audience of one, which is me, so that I can understand what I am sensing and feeling and find words for what I am experiencing—and often, be surprised.

While being a writer attests to some deep-rooted urge to connect, to communicate, to join the conversation, to share, if I put "reader" into the equation while writing, I would be mute.

○

But here I am. I have long had this love, hate, fear relationship with food. Love to eat it when it's delicious and I choose to. Hate the compulsion to keep eating what I don't choose to eat and would rather not; hate feeling uncomfortable when I've stuffed myself full; and hate the binge eating, when anything, even raw Jell-O granules from a packet, will do.

And the fear? Fear of the power food has over me.

And now, I know that I have found liberation.

I am, as I say, living at SFZC. I am a Zen student. I am also a writer. In the right place at the right time?

"To study the Buddha way is to study the self," to quote from a chant we recite, courtesy Zen Master Dogen, the 13th-century Japanese dude who connected with Zen in China then took it back to Japan. Dogen also wrote a set of *Instructions for the Zen Cook*, which is literally about cooking and figuratively about living.

Along with the periods of meditation, lectures and shared chores, meals are at the heart of life here. The *tenzo*, or head of the kitchen, is a Tassajara-trained cook. Tassajara, SFZC's mountain monastery, is renowned for its vegetarian kitchen. The popularity of the Tassajara kitchen led to SFZC opening Greens restaurant at Fort Mason in San Francisco's Marina district in 1979—which to this day serves a constantly evolving menu of some of the most inspired vegetarian and vegan fare available anywhere.

Back at the corner of Page and Laguna, we get fresh produce from Green Gulch Farm, Zen Center's Green Dragon Temple near Muir Beach in Marin, which back then—way before local and seasonal became the norm and Slow Food a trending movement—supplied an in-season organic harvest.

As Zen students we do kitchen prep, like tearing lettuce leaves to fill a huge bowl with bite-size bits. (And watch one exasperated Zen student have a melt-down and toss his "fucking lettuce leaves" over the tenzo.) We do silent *orioke* sessions, which are the formal meals, served in the zendo during sesshins, where you do your darndest to follow a series of stylistic rituals and "just eat" what has been cooked for you, all of it, like it or not, which hypothetically you're not supposed to do (like it, or not like it, that is).

It will be a while before I am given the duty of preparing breakfast for all the temple's residents one day a week. This generally starts with a "sleepless in San Francisco" night because first thing you're going to do before you head for the kitchen is blearily scurry up and down the three floors of passages and past the dorm room in the basement tinkling the little wake-up bell. Imagining not hearing the alarm and failing in this task is an all-night stay-awake and early morning zombie-state recipe.

Then there is the beating of the taiko drum to be done at some point while rushing around the kitchen following the detailed instructions left by the tenzo, be it making sure the grits don't grit or toiling over the tofu, trying to be "present" while anxious that it won't be ready in time. And—are you doing it right? If this all sounds hectic, believe me, it is.

As I say, lots of scope for food and food to scope. And in between, time to wander down to the coffee shop on 16th in the Mission for "moodling—long, inefficient, happy idling, dawdling and puttering," to quote from Brenda Ueland, whose book *If You Want To Write* I spot in The Booksmith in Haight-Ashbury while on a moodling stroll. And am inspired to buy when I pick it up and see pictures of her on the author's page aged 47, which right then is already older than I am, and also aged 91, looking happy and presumably still earning her living "as a writer, editor and teacher of writing."

I carry her with me as my inspiration while what I am uncovering writes itself in my notebooks and on my screen, same as now.

⟳

Back to Helen, the therapist, who is in South Africa.

Post-Paris, post-divorce, I enter a therapy relationship with Helen. I do it after a friend suggests it when she sees me wandering around on New Year's Eve clutching a tequila bottle. It is likely the fifth—or maybe the 15th—New Year's Eve in a row (does *anyone* really like New Year's Eve?) that I have spent in self-created abject misery. Not with someone I like, because I don't know how to be with someone I like.

Helen and I talk consistently through a couple of divorces—hers—while skirting a lot of my real issues. "You are my light relief," she tells me once when she's sick and has postponed all her other clients. Even in therapy, my public face seldom fails me.

In spite of this, we do still engage with a lot of things.

⟳

The hungry mouths analogy comes in reply to a questionnaire I send Helen and around 35 other women. They are an unrepresentative sample in that they are all women I know, some of them vaguely, a few through work, others as close friends.

The questionnaire is about food and sex and masturbation and relationships and being present in the moment and being sensual and more. Things I am puzzling over. My mission when I contact these women, before giving myself a chance to think about how preposterous such inquiries will likely seem and talking myself out of it, is as much to get their thoughts as to see if they think I'm crazy. The overwhelmingly generous and reflective responses tell me they don't (think I'm crazy).

"Aha," Helen the therapist writes back. "You're linking the two hungry mouths: oral and vaginal. I like that."

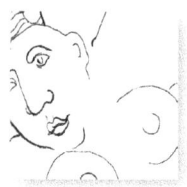

CHAPTER EIGHT

GETTING FORKED

H ow differently might this have turned out?

What's magically morphed into a book project is coming together. It's pre the DIY online publishing era. I don't yet have a green card, so I can't get a job. But I have connected with Media Alliance where I do volunteer tasks, like stuffing envelopes, now presumably an obsolete activity.

And they offer lots of workshops.

I still have the details, cut out and stuck in a file, of the one I sign up for. "How to approach and work with a literary agent," it reads. The instructor is listed as an independent literary agent. It says she is a graduate of the Radcliffe Publishing Procedures Course at Harvard University. When the student is ready, the teacher will appear? I am ready.

It's a three-part class. In the second session, we must submit "an original book proposal for in-class critique and discussion during the third session." In the first session we will get guidelines on said proposal, among other things.

I submit my proposal in session two, having following the instructions issued by the young woman instructor, Karen.

I hand it in with a mixture of enthusiasm and trepidation. It's funny, this writing lark. I am often surprised when I read something I have written, it seems so unfamiliar. This is not because an editor has had a go at it. It's because what appears on the page comes from a mystery place. There's something I want to say. I know what it is, and at the same time, I don't really have a clue.

Then at some point, which may be sooner or later—more often later, and after I've fiddled and I've tweaked—there it is before me. Sort of magical.

Week three, I walk the 30 or 40 minutes to the class, saving on bus fare—and because I love to walk the streets of San Francisco—and take my seat at the large rectangular wooden table in the assigned room.

I don't recall if there was more than the critiques that week. In my memory, the teacher read each person's submission, gave her views on whether the proposal was likely to excite an agent and made suggestions on what, if anything, could make it better.

Not mine, though.

She is going through the class, calling on people, reading their proposals, making comments. But I am waiting. And she doesn't get to me.

I wait, trepidation mounting.

My mind goes from "maybe she's mislaid it" to "Did I put it in the wrong place when she took them from us? No, it must be the subject matter. It must be my ridiculous idea. It's so bad she's not going to give me a turn."

Everybody in the room has had theirs returned to them. She's given her verdict, her comments and a written critique. I feel mortified and exposed.

And then, as I finally sink into myself, she calls my name.

"I've left this proposal for last because I think it's one of the best I've seen in a while," she says. She starts to read it to the class. And my heart starts to pound. I look down, because I cannot look up at her. I am aware of her voice way off in the distance muffled by the pounding that's pounding me. I feel hot. My head feels like it's going to burst.

"It's original, fun, real, sensitive and smart." The words register somewhere off in the distance.

"Your experiences, writing, commitment to self-exploration and sex-positive, food-conflicted women really appeals to me, and to several female editor friends I mentioned this project to."

By now I'm sure I'm about to have a heart attack. I am feeling hugely embarrassed that this is happening. Doing everything I can to hold myself together.

I'm aware that I should be looking at her and acknowledging what she's saying, but I have my head right down almost to the table.

"You have the authority, style and voice to make this a really accessible book to men and women. I think you won't know the exact format until it's written. It strikes me as a mature look at what it means to be feminine now. A greatly needed addition to shelves. Not much politics, just real ideas told honestly. Great work. Again, I truly enjoyed this one!!!!!!!!!!!!!!!"

How do I remember what she said so well, given my stricken state? And why are 15 of a total of 21 exclamation points in this entire book right there?

Because I am copying the words from her written critique that I still have saved in a file.

But right then, when it matters, I simply do not have the capacity to so much as lift my head to look at her; even when she comes and hands my proposal and her comments to me. I know if I try to talk, I will cry, and I will shake, and I will not be able to get any words out. And the background script—"you're going to have a heart attack"—is repeating itself. And "you're ridiculous," maybe the same voice, or another one, is telling me. This voice speaking for the part of me that knows what I ought to be doing. That I should be saying "thank you" and engaging with her and asking her if I can follow up with her. If, seeing she likes my idea, she will be my agent. If I can actualize my book and share my success with her.

I am 41 years old. I know there are people who think of me as successful. I have held down—no, done really well at—some cool jobs; achieved success in many spheres. All the while feeling like a fraud—never like an adult. And right now some familiar default mode has kicked in and I simply cannot do what I know I should and what I'd like to do, any more than I can fly.

I force myself to get up and go through the motions of leaving the room, head still down as if shamed. Feeling ashamed. Of myself.

I catch the bus home to my small room with its single futon, narrow work desk and Tandy laptop. I feel, at the same time, happier and more elated than I have ever felt in my life—and foolish and humiliated.

With the prospect of the 4:45 a.m. wake-up bell followed by the harsh clack, clack, clack of the wooden *han* and the roll of the taiko drum calling us to 5:20 a.m. zazen, the storm subsides.

◯

Ideas have bubbled into my consciousness around eating and living and sex and food and relationships, including the relationship with self. ("You're going traveling *alone*?" someone asks. How about: "No, I'm going with myself," as the reply?)

And in the context of relationships with others, not having a voice, as in being shy.

Have you noticed how many people hang out in pairs and packs? Then there are those who are more often on their own. Or they might be part of the pair or in a pack—but they're feeling separate and cut off. You wouldn't know from the outside. You will know, if this has ever been you.

"Shame," I found written in an old journal: "A feeling of awful self-consciousness that makes us urgently wish we could disappear."

The agent. Why didn't I try to connect with her when sanity returned along with the light of day?

Sure I did. Diligently.

But she went to ground somewhere and never got back.

Do I want food—or do I want sex?

The bonobos, it seems, have it right. Google these small "pygmy chimp" great apes of Central Africa and you'll learn they have a lot of sex.

They have sex to avoid conflict, to show affection, to indicate social status and for stress reduction. They have sex in virtually all partner combinations and in a variety of positions.

The abundant sex is presumed to be a factor in the lower levels of aggression they display, compared with other apes.

Bonobos also have sex before they eat. When they come upon a new food source, the excitement of it will usually lead to communal sexual activity, presumably—I read online—to decrease tension and encourage peaceful feeding.

Sex before food.

Eat to a bloat, you will never feel sexual.

Ever tried sex with a large-bellied lover? Or when your stomach is uncomfortably full? Yes, you can do contortions and work around it. But it's not sexy.

"Sex and food. Food and sex. Embracing, like reluctant Siamese twins. For many women, food and sex have become the intimate coupling and this relationship is the kernel of my book. But to see it as a book about food and sex is to say that food is beef and potatoes served nightly at six and sex is the missionary position when the church bell rings on Sunday."

How do I know this is what I wrote as the introduction to the proposal for the agent when it was written such a long time ago?

Because I still have it in the same file as her critique.

Do I want food—or do I want sex?

In the dining room at SFZC, I play with choosing not to eat when my answer is sex, and instead, allow the sexual feelings to grow and flow. I find it isn't essential that I do anything about these feelings, although I can get into them and enjoy them.

Sometimes I play with breathing deeply and intentionally, following the "in" breath, then the "out" breath, noting the stirring of my sensual nature. In my little room I might put on some music, close my eyes, bend and flex gently, submit my moving body to the rhythms and the beat. Or stretch this way and that, eyes closed, my focus on the muscles and their flow. Or go for a walk; striding out and enjoying the sensuality of my moving body.

I commit to being a truly sensual being in all that I do. Not that I always remember. But, like a meditation, coming back each time I became aware that I am "gone."

There's something reassuringly connecting about experiencing your (my) sensual and sexual nature when sitting down (feeling the butt on the chair, the tensions in the body and letting them go) or standing, walking, shopping, cooking dinner, going to the loo, reading my book (these days sometimes my Kindle), walking in the street noticing the sexuality and sensuality in those I pass—connecting remotely, in a sensual way.

You know how, when a small child is focused on wanting something and is crying for it? If you distract the child with something else, he or she will forget about the first thing and become involved with the second. Not if the child is truly hungry or tired and that's why they're crying. But at other times, with other things.

Well, slowly but surely, the "food or sex" thing works to change the focus in the same way.

As I started doing all this while at the same time paying attention to what I ate, what I thought when I ate, and consciously thinking about food in the context of where it came from, I noticed I could more easily expand my awareness and tune into my body with its complex layers of feelings and desires.

I noted I was eating more thoughtfully—and a lot less.

I noted these things and felt delighted.

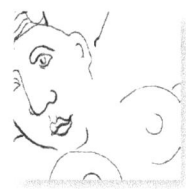

CHAPTER NINE

_____

THE DEVIL MADE ME DO IT

"The greatest gift you can give yourself is to be present."
—Ryushin Paul Haller, Soto Zen roshi, teacher and former abbot,
San Francisco Zen Center

A Catholic nun from Korea needs temp lodgings and comes to stay at SFZC. That she's paying guest student rates means she needs to follow the guest student schedule, which involves meditation. When she learns this requires her to try to empty her mind and simply follow her breath, she confides in her fractured English that she is in a quandary.

She feels she'll be damned if she does (meditate) and damned if she doesn't (pray).

So she goes off to consult her priest—and returns a lot happier. "He said God knows everything, so it's fine. Just sit. No need to pray."

Some time later I interview a born-again Christian woman. The fundamentalist type. The sort who might well have a bumper sticker that reads: "If this car is driverless know that we've been raptured."

Now, while raptured might sound rapturous, as in great sex and profound orgasms, in this context, it is quite the opposite. The first time I heard of this form of rapture was from a hot pro tennis player I dated—just once—because as the evening heated up, after he advised me on the benefits of cold showers to, well, essentially kill passion, he told me his reward for being "good" was that one day he and all the chosen would be raptured, as in zoomed up somewhere, leaving behind, in his case, just an empty pair of tennis shoes. Sort of sexually challenging had the image not been so funny.

What I'm interviewing the Christian woman about has nothing to do with religion. But she brings it up and quizzes me on my relationship with Jesus.

I, in turn, ask if she ever meditates, at which she looks alarmed.

"You must never do that," she warns. "If you empty your mind, the devil will jump straight in."

Empty my mind? Ha. Some hope.

It's early December and I am two days into my first seven-day *sesshin* at SFZC, which means you sit cross-legged on your black cushion in the zendo for a week facing the wall from 5:15 a.m. to whenever after 9:30 p.m. you're released or concede defeat.

Meditation instruction makes it sound so easy. They give the same set of guidelines at the BRC in South Africa, at SFZC, and at a Pema Chödrön-inspired Shambhala group I join when I get my green card and my first American job, writing and editing for a wine magazine, and go live in the historic city of Sonoma, considered the birthplace of winemaking in California. They add 108 prostrations to the mix when I visit the Sonoma Zen Mountain Center, because that's the Korean Zen way. This leaves me gym-workout incapacitated and unable to walk for a week.

At its simplest, you sit tall and straight, ears above shoulders, on your designated cushion (zafu), legs crossed in the manner 100 YouTube videos and who knows how many books can tell you, upright-facing left palm gently resting in upright-facing right palm, thumbs touching (one of many awareness points to bring you back if you drift off), eyes softly focused downward in Zen, lightly closed in other forms (because Buddhism, like Christianity, has many flavors). And then, "you just sit there and breathe normally—nothing special," Antony Osler, the first teacher I took a Zen workshop with, in South Africa, told me.

Oh yes?

Back to day two of my first SFZC sesshin. What I am most clear about at this point is that my mind has a mind of its own and this mind dictates my thoughts, my feelings and, it seems, just about everything else. I don't have a say.

Empty it?

Sounds easy.

But fat fucking chance.

The word that pops up to describe this mind as I journal—which is something I'm not meant to be doing between meditation sessions, but I'm a writer, right?—is recalcitrant.

I know as I sit there that I'm supposed to be in the here and now. In reality I'm almost anywhere and everywhere else.

My inclination is to go and speak to Blanche or to Paul, the priests leading the sesshin, to confess that I'm a fraud. I sit in the upright posture looking still and calm. But it's a lie.

All day my mind has been dancing from problem to problem; solving them, having conversations, making up stories. It has been to South Africa numerous times and told my daughter exactly how she should run her life. When I notice it's skipped off there, I catch it and tell it firmly: "Attend to your own practice."

And I attempt to bring it back. To refocus it on the breath. Consciously to be aware of this breath breathing me.

But in a flash, it's back in South Africa. Now having conversations with the ex-boyfriend. Sure, we didn't have a commitment to maintain our relationship, and sure, I've done a bunk, but to drop the bomb on page three of a letter that someone else has moved in…

At which point I zoom in on the tension in my forehead. "Don't do that. You'll get frown lines and look grumpy," I scold myself and focus, seriously hard, on untensing.

Then it hurtles off again and I watch it grasp and hold forth on this idea, then that idea. Each time, soon as I catch it, I reel it back; back to the breath.

At some point when I catch it, it has alighted on the man sitting on the cushion next to me. I don't know him because he's new—just moved into a room three doors down on the third floor, Page Street side of the building, from mine. I note that because he's nice-looking, my mind keeps endowing him with all manner of agreeable qualities. I see what it's doing and choose not to be taken in, which is just as well because two days later, after he's tried to strike up a conversation several times when during sesshin you're meant to be silent, dammit, and twice, at night, knocked on my door, I've decided he's a creep.

Which prejudice I manage to carry with me and reinforce in one way or another as long as he's living in the building. All the while feeling vaguely curious about him, especially when I hear he's an academic and that he's inviting Zen students to drug conferences and that he's working in a forensic lab cutting up dead bodies. But I hold on to my prejudice even when I hear some people say he's a bit spacey and smiley because he's had a minor stroke and others say it's drugs.

And why the hell won't he shut his door when the Chinese Zen student who succumbs to his advances moves in with him? Because it's discombobulating walking past, given that I don't want to think about what they might be doing in there. Much as I admire her for being comfortable enough to venture naked through the corridors late at night to the women's bathroom.

I kick myself years later when I read that he has been arrested near a decommissioned nuclear missile silo in Kansas—remodeled complete with Jacuzzi, Italian marble tiles and $85,000 audio speakers—and is subsequently sentenced to serve two life sentences without parole for producing 90 percent of the world's supply of LSD in said silo. I read the details in the San Francisco Chronicle. It says one of his letters of support, when seeking clemency, came from a British lord and lady known for trepanation. Holes drilled in skulls to expand consciousness?

Oops. I call myself a journalist and I missed all that.

Back in the zendo, during the afternoon of day two, there is a fleeting window when I feel at one with my breath and the sounds around me and think, like, Wow! I could sit zazen for the rest of my life.

Which means the moment is gone. I'm gone. Back to telling myself to just sit, come back; sit and come back. And soon, long before bedtime, I feel trapped. Ready to get up and run. Escape.

So I force myself to not move. Watch my inclination to bolt. Feel my aching back and tiredness.

Just watching all of it, I notice myself thinking that this zazen replicates how I run my life.

I note that if I am going to complete the book I'm writing, to complete anything I might want to complete, I need to do it like this zazen. Just keep at it, moment by moment, coming back, coming back; note the interruptions, but don't let them have their way with me.

When I go to bed I take three cold capsules to help me breathe as the congestion in my nose isn't helping matters and I want to sleep.

I wake before my 4:30 alarm in ill humor and wonder if this is because I'm seeing the real me and it's not pleasant. Is this what Michael Wenger, the priest who gives a lecture on day three, is talking about when he says we can expect that all our "other selves" and "toxic waste" will come to the fore while sitting? And don't the experts say we should keep a close eye on toxic waste, not hide it out of sight, as it inevitably leaks?

During a brief post-lunch break, I rationalize that while we are advised not to read—same as not to write—I'm sure it's OK to cast an eye over a little Suzuki Roshi, on meditation, for inspiration. I read a story about four kinds of horses: excellent, good, poor and bad. "The best horse will run slow and fast, right and left, at the driver's will, before it sees the shadow of the whip; the second best will run as well as the first one does, just before the whip reaches its skin; the third one will run when it feels pain on its body; the fourth will run after the pain penetrates to the marrow of its bones. You can imagine how difficult it is for the fourth one to learn how to run!"

I feel like the fourth horse trying to do this zazen thing. "The bad horse," the judge-voice says.

Writing in my journal helps me clear out some of the garbage and see it for what it is—in this case, my mind's endless waffling and ramblings that, without distractions, are shoving themselves in my face.

Writing, I get some clarity. I remind myself that all I have to do is keep sitting with the breath and the body, moment by moment, and see what comes up.

Like in an adventure novel?

On day four, in the evening, I think that, just maybe, I have an inkling of a breakthrough.

This comes after noting earlier in the day that I can stay more focused during walking meditation by pretending I'm walking on fake fur; then on velvet; and finally I settle on invoking the imagined sensation of a thin-baked layer of beach sand. The sort you sometimes get on top of the softer sand that's nice to walk barefoot on as it gently cracks.

But when I steel myself to be fully aware during my sitting meditation, I feel the mind squashing the breath, weighing down on it and crowding it out completely.

Then in the last period of zazen, the thought "empty mind" comes to mind, followed by the idea that if I can sort of move the mind outward, this will create a hollow for the breath. I visualize the hollow as a glassy space and conjure up a windowpane, but this doesn't cause it to empty. So I try the image of a clear mirror, as I remember having read about the mind as a mirror.

This doesn't work either.

So then I create a kind of funnel and turn the breath into a sort of balloon that expands in my brain when I breathe in and creates an empty space where the air would be. This way the thoughts and mind things are pushed out of the way.

By the end of it all, I am mentally exhausted. My head is aching. But I feel pleased with myself and look forward to putting my strategy to test in the morning.

I think of asking Paul if I'm on track with my efforts but I hesitate as this all sounds very bizarre, even to me.

I don't know if it is supposed to be so much effort.

I do know I've been told that Zen meditation is about doing nothing other than just breathing normally, or letting the breath breathe you, and lightly following it with awareness, noting thoughts that arise and letting them go. I remember Antony Osler's "nothing special" comment. I've heard that from others too.

And of course anyone who knows anything about meditation will tell you not to do what I was doing. That meditation isn't about mental contortions, being anal and beating yourself up.

On the other hand, going back to that Zen Master Dogen quote, it *is* about studying the self. Which can be a devilishly sobering exercise.

Years later I read a comment in a transcript of an afternoon lecture Suzuki Roshi gave about 25 years before I sat my first sesshin at SFZC. "We always say 'just to sit.' And if you do, you will find out that Zen practice—just to sit—is not easy. Just to sit may be the most difficult thing."

Aha. He knew.

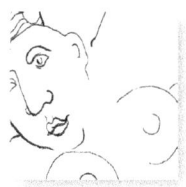

CHAPTER TEN

EGG-STACY

Picture the scene. My first vivid food memory. A string-bean kid about five years old, fair hair braided into two long plaits, alone in the dining room and seated at a large, oval, wood table. The shiny sort you can't put your coffee mug on because it marks.

If someone were to draw the scene for a comic book and suspend a thought-bubble above the girl's head, the bubble would be dark, brooding, and contain a single word. "Angst."

I am sitting over my plate trying to avoid the stare of this big fried egg that's peering up at me—an imposing ocher iris with a blotch of blood right in the middle suggesting a shriveled red pupil. The egg is daring me to eat it. My stomach is also daring me to eat it, so that it might revolt and throw up.

Meanwhile, my father has dared me not to eat it.

Looking back, my childhood seemed haunted by eggs. I can still see my small Scots grandmother, sent to a relative in South Africa as a young girl after both her parents died—her trademark silver widow's peak unflinching under its daily hand-job coating of Lux toilet soap and her bunions ("Spanish onions") squeezed into a pair of size three pointy-toed high-heeled pride-feels-no-pain pumps—chasing after me with an egg flip. This was her way of disguising raw eggs to make them marginally more palatable.

She would dollop a couple of tablespoons of fine baker's sugar and half a teaspoon of vanilla essence into two yolks, separated and dropped into her favorite Pyrex bowl. As she beat, the thickening mixture would turn a creamy yellow.

In a second bowl she would whip the whites, plus another tablespoon of sugar, into stiff mounds. She would lightly fold her two concoctions into a glass and present me with what she disingenuously called a milkshake.

My father knew how to suck eggs. Raw ones, through toothpick-sized holes he would pierce on the pointy sides in the shell. This sucking feat reliably made both my mother and me gag. Fortunately, when he was doing breakfast, he gave me my eggs cooked. Only this particular day, I didn't feel even slightly fortunate. He had cooked me an egg for breakfast—and whatever he cooked, it was my duty to eat. He was a Pole who'd come to South Africa after World War II looking for meaning and purpose. My mother and I were what he got. He had a tendency to grunt and shout, probably in a futile attempt to make himself understood in his non-native English, which struck me about a month after I got to San Francisco.

○

The location is a therapist's office in Marin county, California. I'm there with the friend I came to join in San Francisco and the boyfriend who didn't want me to come. But he's not dumb. For a brief period after I get there, until the wheels fall off between my friend and me, he knows he has to act like he accepts me to have a hope in hell of keeping her even vaguely placated.

Who we've come to see is his business therapist. He also, I have learned, has a personal therapist; a therapist he goes to with his two young children from the ex-wife; and a relationship therapist he drags my friend along to because she's decided she made a mistake leaving her South African husband, who has refused to have her back. As one might expect, this new guy's ego is seriously at stake and he needs all the help he can get.

This includes his sweat lodges and men's groups. Maybe other things too. I don't remember.

I do remember feeling like I'd walked in on the California cliché. Or a wanna-be Woody Allen movie. (Too much drama; too little humor; mediocre script.)

This day's therapy session, reading between the lines, is to have the therapist try to persuade my friend to see the wisdom of her boyfriend's ways—at least in terms of what he feels she should do to support his business.

The therapist's intention, he tells us, is to give us each equal time to share thoughts and feelings, the plan being to gather good ideas. Fair enough.

Except had he asked, I could have saved him time.

My friend, since forever, meaning all the years I've known her, is only interested in being heard.

So, as the poor man attempts to guide the session, she gets louder.

As he persists, she gets louder still.

Eventually, as she endeavors to have her say and not to hear, her voice is all that's in the room. Voice as in piercing noise; no discernible words.

At that moment I think of my father.

Then I remember him telling a story to an ex-boyfriend (of mine) about his ladder being stolen from where it was tied to a drainpipe outside.

I remember the boyfriend saying, "That's nice."

I remember asking this boyfriend afterwards what was so fucking nice about my dad having had his ladder stolen.

I remember this boyfriend saying, "I never understand a word your father says."

I remember being amazed as I had never heard an accent. But clearly, others did.

You speak. You want to communicate. You expect to be heard.

If you can't speak out when you want to, as comes with painful shyness, there's a tendency to withdraw. To become depressed. If you can speak out and you're not heard, you'll most likely shut the fuck up—or shout. Flight or fight? My dad shouted.

Beyond my dad's accent, people would have heard the shouting. Been scared. As I sometimes was.

Back in Marin, the therapist concedes defeat and ends the session.

My friend's boyfriend gives me his car keys. He says he will drive home with my friend in her car (his, really).

He suggests I drive south across the Golden Gate Bridge then keep going. I'll find a nice stretch of coastline and some interesting little towns.

I do—and I do. But I turn back when I reach Santa Cruz; too stressed out to find a parking spot and go exploring, both by the therapy session and the driving, for the first time in the U.S. and on the right side of the road, which in the world I've left behind is the wrong side.

I stop on the journey back at a roadside diner in Davenport where I sit and cry into my hamburger sensing that a friendship is disintegrating and my new-career plans and general plans for the U.S. are unravelling.

⟳

Back to the scared kid at the table. Back to me and my dad. Back to my deep knowing that if the egg remains on my plate, the gathering black cloud will weigh heavier and heavier with the thunder of his rage.

It must have been about then that a very large book magically called to me from its spot in the second to bottom shelf of the dining room bookcase. When my father next leaves the room, I tippy-toe across to it, quiet as a mouse and quick as a blink, hoist it onto the table next to my plate, open it somewhere near the center, slide my egg onto the left-hand page, gingerly close the book over the egg, return it to the bookcase. And hearing my father's heavy tread, sit back down before my plate.

Hot with guilt and stiff with fear, I wait for him to guess what I have done. Instead, he showers me with gruff praise.

I expect he was so overjoyed at winning the contest, he forgot to wonder how I had moved my egg from plate to mouth without leaving a trace of yolk.

Whatever happened to the egg? I don't know.

I peeked at that book often and for many months when I thought nobody was looking, terrified to eyeball it straight on in case my gaze propelled someone else to look.

And also, I was afraid of what I might see because in my mind, the egg eventually turned a violent shade of blue. The moldy blue mess grew many legs. And one day these moldy legs jumped down from the bookcase and, carrying the book, walked right out the house.

The thing is, one day the book simply was not there. It had disappeared. A new book was in its place. Who found it and what became of it remains a mystery as nothing was ever said.

⟡

We all have our individual food stories. They can involve time and place and sometimes people we love.

My father. He had traveled the world on ships before settling in South Africa. I thought of him as adventurous and exotic. He was also, in many ways, uncompromising and remote. Except when it came to food. It was his passion. His hobby. His obsession. His way of expressing love.

And it was serious business.

He cooked. Beef stroganoffs, pavlovas, zabagliones, borschts, potato pancakes, goulashes, prawns grilled to perfection, dumplings, tripe dishes, chicken soup for the soul…

He cooked in the old-fashioned way, heavy on butter and cream. His repertoire was international and limitless. You ate. If you had seconds, he gave a rare smile.

Fast-forward going-on four decades. I am living at the San Francisco Zen Center. Not so very long after moving in, during a dinner, I catch myself having seconds and hesitate long enough to ask: Why am I about to force-feed myself when I am full?

In a flash, I realize I am still having seconds for my father. Which isn't doing either of us any good, given that my poor body needs a respite, not a refuel—and he, at the time, has been dead for eight long years.

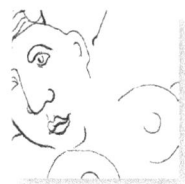

CHAPTER ELEVEN

DYING FOR IT

Ponder these.

If you knew you had just weeks to live, what would you do that you're not doing now?

What would you prioritize?

Are there things waking you up worried and obsessing?

Fast-forward to your last night on earth. The end is nigh.

Thinking back to now, from there, is this how you want to be spending your time?

These are coaching questions that can help one weigh priorities, make decisions, inspire new perspectives.

The first time I spend the morning at SFZC, having found the place during the week and been told by a grumpy man called Gerald that I should come back on Saturday for the formal public program, the talk is on death and dying.

We sit virtually on top of one another squashed together in the tatami-matted Buddha Hall on round black cushions. The speaker is Frank Ostaseski. He tells us about SFZC's residential care facility—home of the Zen Hospice Project of which he is founding director—just down the street. He talks about some of the HIV/AIDS and cancer patients who have lived and died there. And he speaks at length about the Zen Hospice Project's volunteer training program, which is taking applications.

I feel I've died and gone to heaven. Sounds funny, even to me, given that if you quizzed me on this, I'd tell you I think the only version of heaven that comes with a guarantee are heavenly moments experienced right here on earth, and before we kick the bucket. And that we need not get stuck in hellish times.

○

My Polish dad worked hard and asked for very little from me. He asked that I eat what he cooked and enjoy it. He asked that I get an education—"they can't take that away from you" was the mantra I grew up with. And he asked to die in his own bed. He didn't specifically ask this of me, but I knew.

One morning when he was 74 and had been home sick for a while, but convinced he'd return to work, the doctor said he needed to go to hospital and called an ambulance to fetch him.

He flayed in a semi-delirious way, trying to fight off the men who strapped him to the stretcher to carry him down the three flights of stairs. Watching, I was torn. I was super-aware of the "own bed" request. I didn't know these were death throes. If I had, would I have done anything different? What? I felt helpless and useless. You're expected to love your parents. This is not to say you have to *like* them. But I liked my dad. His adventurous past. His worldly aura. His generosity and loyalty. His dependability and stoicism. I liked that I knew he really liked me. My dad is the reason I think that, to this day, I like men. And if I could wave a wand, would rather be one.

It's funny, really, because my dad and I—we never had an honest-to-goodness conversation. The relationships in our tiny family were complex. My mom had made me her confidante when I was 10. My mom's "forever" mantra was "Don't tell your father."

So I watched him go.

And was left with years of guilt because he died that night. In a horrible cold ward in a large government hospital among strangers.

I was finally, some years later, while in therapy with the aforementioned Helen, able to let the guilt go. She suggested I write a letter to my father explaining all I'd like to have said and done and told him and not been party to. I was then to burn it in a candle flame.

Being of lazy disposition and not too touchy-feely, I made up the letter in my head and burned it in my head, too. And the catharsis was amazing. Not least because the brain doesn't distinguish too much between what it thinks and "hard reality," which anyway, is all made up. And if you want to read more about that from a non-Buddhist practical stance, read *The Art of Possibility* by Boston Philharmonic conductor Benjamin Zander and his psychotherapist wife Rosamund Stone Zander.

◯

My father, meanwhile, in death, left me two profound gifts. The first was hard-hitting, in-the-face tangible—yet at the same time, intangible. And it still makes me ponder. It came about after the hospital called to say he was dead, and did we want to see the body? We drove down, dazed and confused. Is death ever not a shock?

And there he was.

But at the same time, he wasn't.

There was a body, but "he" was gone. Switched out. Extinguished. No more.

Gone out—or gone where? Who knows? But I do know that it was no more my father in death than—what?—James Bond? The Polish Pope? The Holy Ghost? Monty Python's dead parrot?

The second thing he left me was tangible—in a different way. I had hated how helpless I felt being with my father in his dying. That I'd escaped into my work and been useless in the preceding weeks bothered me hugely. I wanted to connect with this dying thing. I might have bombed out on my dad but I surely didn't need to bomb out on my friends. So that first morning at SFZC was like the gift I'd been waiting for.

◯

And the gifts of the Zen hospice training and working with those who came there for a period that might be short, or sometimes longer, were multitudinous. And time spent with them was uplifting, not depressing: being there with the intention of answering to their needs, doing your best to honor their requests. ("Please sing to me," an Asian lady with cancer, thin as a plucked sparrow, asks me during my first shift. Jeez, with my voice? But a lullaby comes from somewhere and self-consciously I sing—and she drifts off to sleep.) Each of them, though "officially" dying, living fully, in their own way, right up until the final breath.

The folk running the program stressed self-care at the monthly support meetings for volunteers. We were told to become aware of what topped us up and fueled us and to be sure to add lots of it, which might be music or dancing or, I am sure, lovemaking, even if nobody talked about that.

This focus on sensual feel-good practices, and feeding the spirit, informed not just my life and my interactions with the hospice residents, but also the new habits I was developing, across the street at SFZC, around food.

◠

And let me stress that this was not about denying and avoiding dark places. On the contrary, sometimes they're unavoidable. And they can heighten the pleasures of the flip side. And living in fear of them can reduce the possibility of a rich, full and well-lived life.

◠

When I got my first American green card job, working as an editor on a wine lifestyle magazine in Napa, I moved out of SFZC and went to live in the town of Sonoma.

My one option for a meditation group to join was to drive way up a mountain near Glen Ellen to the Sonoma Zen Mountain Center, which I did—rarely—in my little old Nissan Sentra purchased from Sonoma Bob, the local car dealer, who was elderly, walked with difficulty, but went country dancing four nights a week and liked to tell his dance partners: "If you feel old age creeping up on you, it's me."

My other option was to stroll across the plaza to the Shambhala Center, which was a Pema Chödrön sitting group.

Here, there were good people, good *genmaicha*—brown rice (popcorn) green tea—and pretty regularly, a scary "dark place" Tibetan Buddhism meditation practice called Tonglen that if you persisted, slowly but surely, was uber-liberating.

It's a guided meditation, although when you've done it a few times (there are YouTube videos) you can guide yourself.

You start off by bringing to mind people you like and showering them with (happy) golden light. Then, at some point, you're asked to call to mind someone or something you don't like (or that scares you). You breathe in all the darkness—then breathe out showerings of (lustrous) golden light. You take in suffering—then breathe out happiness and good vibes. Really difficult at first. But you keep going deeper into darkness.

The world doesn't end.

In fact, living in it starts to feel better.

When you need to confront your own dark places you may find you're less inclined to opt for safety, driven by fear. Or to want to run away.

You may find yourself better able to open yourself to love and its bedfellows, risk and hurt.

Susan Jeffers wrote a great book many years ago called *Feel the Fear...and Do It Anyway*. This practice helps with the "do it anyway."

One-and-a-half years into a job on the Oakland Tribune copydesk, a convergence of events made me lose my grip and start down the slippery slide to where a physical depletion of some joy-chemical seems to occur. At least that's what it feels like.

The paper was laying people off. I was hating my job—taking sick days, which I'd never done. Usually work had been my escape during desolate times. Now work had become the ogre. I would look out the window of the apartment I was sharing with my then-boyfriend and see the Tribune Tower building where I was due to start at 2 p.m. It developed the beheading aspects of the Tower of London.

I spoke to the editor, not to actually spell out that I was depressed, because who wants to admit to that? But I told him I was unhappy. They were doing more layoffs. I asked to please be on the list. He suggested I see the company's independent therapist, so I did.

Sitting literally knee to knee in a tiny room across from Lake Merritt, telling him my issues that seemed boring even to me, the guy—nodded off. Out, like a light. Disconcerting, if pretty funny. And not the reason I finally saw no option other than to resign.

Then, feeling desperate, and as a Kaiser medical plan member, I made an appointment with someone in their psych section. She didn't fall asleep. Instead, I found myself placed on disability for major recurring depression. After the fact, even though I'd resigned, she wrote a letter and formally laid me off from my old job.

Which is how I ended up at some industrial court place in downtown Oakland, my Japanese American Francophile best California friend, Meg, in tow for support, pleading my case before a labor court officer. Opposing my appeal for job termination benefits were the editor, someone from the newspaper group's HR department and a company legal person. My depression, my unexpected savior at Kaiser, a letter from the dozy therapist and fessing up to and confronting my "shame" won out.

And this was the crucial turning point—because I was advised to attend Kaiser's group cognitive therapy depression classes. While I had known it came down to the thinking—my thinking—they gave the nitty gritty stuff.

The final nail was hammered into my depression coffin a couple of years later so that now if the slippery slope so much as blips on the horizon, I'm outta there. When writing a grant proposal for funding to continue a series of successful depression and mindfulness workshops at SFZC, I came across research on staying present and riding depression's waves; on eschewing brooding and disengaging from negative thoughts when they pop up (whew—what relief); on neuroplasticity; on becoming aware and becoming free.

I don't dispute that there are times for depression meds and people who need them, but there are also tools—and there is mindfulness.

And when I think about that coaching question: "Fast-forward to your last night on this earth. Is this how you want to have spent your time?"

Categorically not wallowing in depression. I've wasted enough time there.

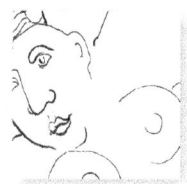

CHAPTER TWELVE

INTERRUPTUS

"There is nothing about my body that I like," Nina, a super-successful, extremely attractive and neither fat nor even pleasantly plump 50-year-old tells me during a coaching session when we are talking about her sensuality, which, she said, she had excised from her life.

"I cannot be sensual until I lose weight and go to a gym and tone. And that means I can't get a sex life either. I mean, look at these legs!" she laments.

"Can you think of one good thing about your legs?" I ask.

"My knees are too big. My legs are pasty. I don't bother to shave them in winter because—who's going to see them?" she replies.

Nina is married. But, she's said, the marriage is on the rocks. No sex in "well, maybe twice in the past four years there's been an attempt, but he's not interested and I've long lost interest."

"Can you just pick out one good thing? Say, about the legs," I persist, still focusing on them because they're what came up.

"No. I just don't like them," she says.

"Don't they benefit you in any way?" I implore.

"Well, I suppose they get me around," she relents. "But that doesn't mean I like them."

"So, what about your arms?" I ask.

"They remind me how old I am and how much time I spent in the sun when I was younger," she says. "And don't try and push me to find something good about them! If I had a boob lift, lost 10 pounds and got into shape, I might start to like myself. Then I might start to feel sensual. Then I might get divorced and focus on getting a sex life."

"What is it like to walk around all day carrying something you dislike so intensely?" I ask.

"I just don't think about it," she says.

So what if Nina (not her real name) was pointing out these same limitations but directing the comments to a friend? Verbal abuse?

We hate bullies. But what about when we bully ourselves?

○

"I've come to pitch a story on life coaching."

The wine country magazine that gave me my first green card job in the United States has folded. The "senior" magazine I worked on in Emeryville has folded. I am now the editor of a glossy lifestyle mag based in the San Francisco East Bay town of Walnut Creek. And I have never heard of life coaching.

"What's that?" I ask. The freelancer sitting in my office tells me about a local woman who never took a day off work and whose company was floundering. Now the woman is living a

Tim Ferriss *4-Hour Workweek* lifestyle, coining the bucks, and she attributes it to the life coach she hired.

I'm not convinced, but this is a good writer and she is willing to write for our rates, so I say: "OK. Make sure you have some coaching sessions yourself, and go for it."

⟳

When I read her story, which I edit myself because I am curious, I think, "Wow, this makes sense. I want to get one, and I want to be one." I start looking at schools.

Three-and-a-half years later, I've done the prerequisite courses, worked with a coach and completed certification with its required 100 paid coaching hours. I have also had, and left, two more jobs and decided that formal employ in the U.S. and I are somehow not a good fit.

So now I have to market myself.

⟳

Everyone says go give talks. In theory the idea excites me. In practice, I cringe at the prospect. So I try sending e-mails. I set up a coaching website. I do a newsletter blast. I get clients by lucky connections and word of mouth. But not enough.

Finally I succumb. Send a proposal to talk at Experience Unlimited, an unemployment resource I've previously connected with between jobs. Endure huge angst trying to write a life-changing, inspiring speech. Suffer through giving it. After which a man comes up to me and says: "Most people, you know, didn't hear you, because you weren't speaking into the mic. And for a talk like that you really should speak to people, not at them. Have you heard of Toastmasters?"

Of course I have. And tried many "get over yourself" things over many years including signing on for lessons with a drama prof, which saw me striding around her living room for several weeks reciting a planned talk. Then literally melting into a waterfall of sweat when I finally gave it.

Now I go home and Google Toastmasters. The closest group to the historic Cleveland Cascade stairs on Lake Merritt in Oakland, just across from where I'm living, is Rockridge Toastmasters. They meet once a week, from 7 p.m. to 8 p.m., across the lake in the Veterans Memorial Building.

○

My experience with the book agent might have been life-changing had I been a different—functioning—person. But I have no idea my first time at Toastmasters, listening to an architect speak so nervously and hesitantly that it makes me think I can fit in here, exactly how transformative this will be.

○

So here I am, eight years old and on holiday from boarding school. I am quiet; an introvert. My friend, Diane, is talkative and extrovert. She is going to be an actress. I don't know what I am going to be, but definitely not an actress. In fact, we will both end up as journalists.

"We're going to do a play," Diane says one day. Diane lives with her parents and brother at the hotel my father manages, goes to school across the street, and has friends. She is even allowed to have a bicycle. My mother says a bicycle is dangerous. She says when I was given a scooter, at age two, I whooped "Look at me!"—then fell on the handlebar and knocked out my front teeth.

"We're going to do *Alice in Wonderland*." Diane has clearly thought it all through. "We'll invite the hotel guests, sell them tickets and give the money to charity." The hotel has a residential block and several permanents. "We'll do it on the veranda of the annex," Diane continues as, meeting no resistance, she warms to her plan and her acquiescing collaborators.

The annex has a large tiled porch with pillars out front and a single step down to grass. "We'll put out chairs and use sheets for curtains." Not a problem. All our beds have sheets.

Besides me, she assigns roles to three or four other children. I don't remember them by name and I don't recall much about Diane's *Alice* story, except that she wrote a script and said I would be Alice and must wear an Alice band in my hair.

She tells us how to arrange the stage and finds bricks and makes a circular rabbit hole. We string up the sheets that we pull from our beds, put out chairs that we drag from the rooms, invite whatever elderly residents Diane can coerce, and charge them the fee she says is right.

The sheets open and Diane tells me to get on stage. I make my entrance—and then it happens. I freeze. Not a word comes out of my mouth. I try to say what I'm meant to. I really want to. I will the words to come out. But all I can do is stand and stare at the small audience staring at me.

I hear Diane, from the side, prompting me, her stage whisper getting louder as the seconds tick by. After an eternity, I hear her say "get down the rabbit hole; get down the rabbit hole." And that's it. She takes over my lines. Wonderland continues without Alice.

Afterwards, Diane counts the money and divides it equally among us. "This isn't enough for charity," she decides, then leads us off to Alexandra Park, where she and I would sometimes go and climb trees. At the park is a cricket oval and grandstand, a circular covered bandstand and near to that, a store where we spend the money on candy.

And that scenario? Bar the money and the candy and Diane, it repeats itself with tedious regularity. There's Wanda—willful, capable and independent. All on the inside. And then there's Alice—taciturn to the verge of autistic, self-conscious, insecure and angst-riddled. Action-babe versus mealy-mouthed arsehole mute. Wanda with ideas; Alice making sure they're stillborn. Their war for domination—really liberation—defines my life. At high school, feigning a sore throat when asked to read out my essays. As a post-grad college student, hating myself more and more all year as no amount of determination will get a word out of my mouth in class discussions.

Meanwhile, Diane never held my failure in her show against me. In fact, she never mentioned it. And for me, to talk about it would have been to admit that it had happened.

So for years I didn't. Until I shared it as my icebreaker at Toastmasters. Specifically, at Rockridge Toastmasters—an eclectic, diverse group where I made some of the best friends I have in California.

No magical wand was involved in turning me into a normal person able to stand up and speak without shaking, quaking and sweating. It was, plain and simply, getting up, week after week, for four years; repetition being key. And I know I was lucky to land at this particular Toastmasters club that was big-time supportive of individual differences and quirks.

About three years into Toastmasters, through life coaching, I discover Lee Glickstein's Speaking Circles. Had I chanced upon a less fun Toastmasters club not as tolerant of eccentricities, Speaking Circles' no-performance "relational presence" approach would have been my pick—to forge new synapse pathways, rewrite my personal story, become someone I could like.

And while practice did not make perfect, as in turn me into a raving extrovert, all I have to do if I need to speak in public and feel that old default-mode flutter, is remind myself that I have done so, often, and I can.

From this place of freedom I can now see that my compulsive eating and my depression were both tied in with my social phobia and not having a voice. Each needed to be addressed individually and all had to be addressed jointly.

Transforming into someone able to speak out and speak up "in the world" was key.

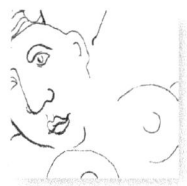

CHAPTER THIRTEEN

THE BIG O

Dateline: San Francisco, August 10, 2013.
Event: "The biggest OM circle in history."

OM? Orgasmic meditation. I first read about it when I'm doing research to write a Sunday magazine feature story on slow sex—erotic, companionable, focused, lazy, satisfying—these terms having been evoked by watching lions having sex.

I am in South Africa for a few months. Family stuff. A friend has invited me for the weekend to his game lodge. While out on a game drive, we come upon this lion and lioness. From our vehicle we watch him approach her, nuzzle a bit, mount her briefly with a reverberating purring growl; at which point she pulls away and flops down, stretches and yawns. He sprawls too, stretches and yawns. They both get up, walk a little way together, flop down, stretch and yawn again. She raises herself, wanders to a different spot. He follows. He nuzzles her again. Mounts her again.

And so it goes. They have four of these brief encounters with us following in our four-wheel drive. Our guide says the pair have been at it in this fashion for a week.

Lion sex. How cool. Imagine a week of slow, erotic, companionable, focused, lazy, satisfying lion sex with someone you really, really like. And OK, I know I'm anthropomorphizing. A male friend goes so far as to admonish me for calling it sex. "Lions don't have sex, they mate," he says.

But I like my lion sex fantasy. Sometime, someone, somewhere...

＊

As I say, an editor—who has been running a series on slowing down trends—has asked me to write an article on slow sex. I have my lion encounter. Then a book pops up in Google called *Slow Sex: The Art and Craft of the Female Orgasm.* I read that its author, San Francisco-based Nicole Daedone, is a long-time Zen student. I learn that her company, called OneTaste, champions orgasmic living. That it is focused on women having more orgasms. That she (through OneTaste) is creating an orgasm movement.

I find a TED talk where she explains the origins of OMing and how she was first OMed, at a party.

I learn that OM is a 15-minute timed practice. It involves the woman getting naked from the waist down and lying with her legs butterflied in a specific way. The man—typically not a boyfriend, but a bloke who has been trained in OM—then sits down next to her, fully dressed. He looks intently at her pussy—OneTaste's preferred terminology—and describes what he sees.

He then, using his index finger, vinyl or latex glove optional, slowly and deliberately and availing himself of lubricant "and no more firmly than you would stroke your eyelid" strokes her clitoris in a prescribed way. I establish that orgasm in OM terms need not necessarily mean climax, but perhaps ripples of intensity, because the focus of the woman being OMed is on being present with what's happening. Not on trying to perform, to please, or to measure herself to some standard. There is some brief feedback dialogue between the woman and the man to end the OM session.

Online, I read Daedone's Turned On Woman's manifesto, which says: "She wasn't always comfortable, but no one can say she didn't enjoy her life."

It ends: "She was courageous. She was turned on."

To rewind. When I get my visa and buy my ticket to San Francisco for a year that will extend to "forever"—which could well be a Zen euphemism for now, then, plus future impermanent permanence—I commit to being celibate for the year. It's a decision grounded in self-preservation. Deeply angst-filled relationships have taken their toll. I am afraid: of my emotions and of myself when my desires hook me into someone and at some deep reptilian brain level, something goes "glob." It's like a form of imprinting takes place and the individual gets gifted with a range of singular qualities that, time may reveal, are singularly absent.

This doesn't happen with all the men I date. It is inevitably men I find attractive to begin with, who then pursue me, and—key—with whom I have good orgasms.

Case in point. These sexy forearms walk into the newsroom one morning, attached to hands I see a bit later typing up a two-fingered frenzy—and I'm done. Or undone.

When I see him walking at a 45 degree drunken lurch the next Friday evening after a bunch of us go to the pub, I see the lurch. But I don't.

Several years later, after break-ups and increasingly more debilitating and less passionate make-ups, a therapist—same Helen—quizzes me on why I want to be in a relationship with an alcoholic. I hear her, but dismiss the words.

Finally a friend says, "Come to Al-Anon." A woman, a stranger, comes up to me after we've shared what's brought us there. She says, "I will get down on my knees and beg you to leave him." She recommends a book called *Don't Help*. I read it—and wake up.

I am finally ready to see. To un-imprint.

Not so simply, though.

My entire body feels raw, like the nerves are inflamed and exposed. My mind goes over and over what I could have done differently. It angsts that he will be happy with someone else. I sleep hugging an old jacket he's left behind for comfort in my misery. Someone told me once that the best way to get over a man is to get under another. But it doesn't work that simply. To start off, you have to meet the right other to get under, which is never a given.

"The mind is like a stage magician…" Tibetan Buddhist Yongey Mingyur Rinpoche says in his book *The Joy of Living: Unlocking the Secret and Science of Happiness*. "It can make us see things that aren't really there."

That's no lie.

So, sure, I will quite happily do things like share a room in Venice with five young male students, met while disembarking at the train station, who tell me they're looking for a sixth person—to get dorm room rates. And go stay in an apartment in Paris with a couple I meet on the train who invite me five minutes after we strike up a conversation and I get a good feeling. And say "Yes" to some Murano factory owner whose name I don't know and who asks if he can fetch me in his motorboat and take me for dinner. And then, when I take my daughter backpacking around Europe for three-and-a-half months when she's 13, we sleep at times on beaches and at train stations and on the ship's deck, crossing from Brindisi, and we hitch-hike through the Black Forest and the Alps and have more than our share of adventures involving strangers.

But while traveling on my own—and in fact on all of the above trips—I note that I never drink enough to get drunk and my body shuts down. Even if I meet someone I like, it's like I'm wearing an invisible chastity belt with a lock.

This physical "safety net" has "just happened" in the past. Unsolicited. Protective.

This time, on going to San Francisco, it's a choice. I don't want to imprint on someone and lose myself when I am on the other side of the world. It's not what I'm going there for.

As I said before, I don't imagine just what this commitment to being celibate will crack open in me. I am not anticipating that it will allow me to develop better relationships with men.

That I'll come to see hunky men as people, not sex objects—and not feel a sex object myself when uninvited solicitations come. Which they do.

"I want to sleep with you because I've never slept with a white South African." This comes from an African American man I have chatted to a couple of times at Angelina's coffee shop in the Avenues in San Francisco, a few blocks from where I live in a basement apartment my first three months in California. He's talked about a girlfriend. He's talked about a heart problem. I thought "how nice" when he suggested an evening stroll. I am more than a little stunned at his off-the-wall out-the-blue unanticipated suggestion.

I feel liberated when I say, "I'm being celibate." I find I can listen to his reprimand that "you must use it or you'll lose it" with interest and no emotional investment.

There are many incidents like this. Being celibate, I feel no pressure to accommodate or to make excuses. Is it that my socialization that told me to comply is being challenged?

○

I like being celibate. But I don't like not having orgasms.

Lucky for me Good Vibrations, then still the original woman-owned sex shop, is a walk through the Mission from SFZC. They have a sign that says, "If you want a job well done, do it yourself." Interesting for a virgin do-it-yourselfer.

At Good Vibes they have people who will answer your timid questions; they even have a room (long gone) where you can try out some of their toys. The Hitachi Magic Wand is still proving its versatility, currently being used by a guy-friend with good effect to treat muscle spasms.

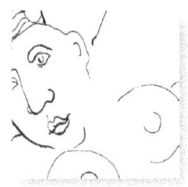

CHAPTER FOURTEEN

MASTER STROKE

Back to August 10, 2013.

I take BART from Oakland, get off at Civic Center and walk fast, just because I like to. I am not familiar with the venue of "the biggest OM circle in history" but have Googled it—the Regency Center—and find it at Sutter and Van Ness.

I feel like a mixing bowl of reticence, curiosity—and resolve: not to let my head have its way with consternation and self-doubt. I have shared with only one person where I'm going because what does one say? I'm going to participate in a group orgasm? I'm going to a kind of conference where conceivably—no, presumably—some stranger will stare deep into my naked pussy, comment on its colorations and curves, then using his index finger slowly and deliberately, and availing himself of lubricant, "and no more firmly than you would stroke your eyelid," involve himself with my clitoris to bring forth orgasm?

All of this in the company of many other women I don't know from Adam (or more aptly, Eve) also gathered here to be stimulated to orgasm by men they don't necessarily know.

Men who will remain fully clothed and focused, not on their own orgasm, but on mine, or, taking into account that this is a group shebang with many women, ours.

Even to me it sounds a little weird. In fact more like unreal, if even possible. At the very least, it is an unusual way to be spending a Saturday.

○

I remember at high school how much I hated being a virgin. Not that anybody talked about things like this. Not to me, anyway. So I simply decided that every other girl in the class had done it. Except maybe Sandra, with the sweaty hands. Although she was quieter than me so thinking back, maybe she was doing it the most, given that it can be easier if you're shy to have sex than to talk.

What sweet relief, then, to return to boarding school after one particular free Sunday—a couple of Sundays each term we were allowed to go home—knowing that he and I, me and the guy I was going out with, had done it too. On the narrow steel divan in my bedroom. Not earth shattering. But he got all shuddery and it felt pretty good.

And whew. There are some burdens to be relieved of.

I feel a little embarrassed and left out not having done certain other things I'd like to be able to say I've done, like cocaine and LSD. Except I have no desire to do them.

But virginity. That was a biggie.

○

As I say, I'd written a feature article that included references to OneTaste and Nicole Daedone from far away on the southern tip of Africa for my story on slow sex. I had signed up for their e-mail list and read a bunch of stuff. Pleasure deficit disorder was the official terminology. That women were stressed out and out of touch with their bodies was the reality.

Sure thing.

All around, I heard women talking about sex—or more pertinently, not having sex. Too fat. Too fucked (as in tired, which was the only fucked some women, notably those stuck on the multitasking treadmill, reported they got). Too busy. Not interested in the guy they had, who they didn't like too much but were too comfortable to leave. No guy available. This, from both younger women and older women. I heard it in coaching sessions, I read it in articles, it came up in general conversations with friends.

"Please write an article and tell men they don't need to be afraid of having to have sex," a divorced woman in her late fifties says. "I meet these men, my age range, and they won't ask me out because they think I'll expect them to be able to get it up and they're scared they'll look foolish. But you know, I don't care. I just want closeness and companionship."

⟡

I have my printout confirming my Day Two attendance at the first Orgasmic Meditation Conference. When I check in, a young woman wearing a Powered by Orgasm T-shirt says since I've never been OMed, I must go for orientation.

In an upstairs room about 30 of us, men and women, are told the OM protocol. A key point is that you can ask anyone to OM you and they are at liberty, for any reason or no reason, to say yes or to say no. In turn, anyone can offer to OM you and ditto, you can accept or decline.

I find myself observing this mixed bag of people and wondering who I might ask. And would I really? And no, better not ask him. Too young. And not that one because he looks (oops, I try to censor my judgments). And not that one because—yikes, scary.

And beyond the flash judgments that arise and make me feel truly mean-spirited, I know I don't want to ask anyone who maybe is not experienced, and who won't do it properly, whatever properly is.

Most things are covered at the briefing so I just ask a couple of bland information-gathering questions when one of the group leaders asks me if I have any.

And then I go and sit in on some break-out sessions on OMing and relationships and a presentation by the hot chick from Rutgers University orgasm lab who talks about all the good things they're finding via MRI when they monitor brain activity during OM stroking sessions, plus the benefits of the "happy hormone" oxytocin that's released, and so forth.

Then I bump into the same young man who was answering questions at the orientation. He asks me how it's going. I ask him, probably rather beseechingly, if I can really just go and ask anyone to OM me, and how do I know who to ask?

He says, "Would you like me to OM you?" I say, "Yes please."

So off he goes and gets me a "nest" number. Then he asks if I have lube, which is for sale in the on-site OM store, and I say no, should I get some? And he says he will, and I should go find my nesting spot for the huge midday OMing session and he will join me there. So I do—and see, glancing around, that the women are all undressing from the waist down. So I do this too, before he arrives and takes his spot on his zafu and tells me how to butterfly my legs using the pillows provided.

And I very consciously do my best to block out the voice in my head that wants to become concerned about my pussy and whether it will look OK as I lie there like a lamb to the slaughter or would that be a butterflied fillet? And he tells me what he sees and proceeds to engage with my clitoris, checking in every so often that I'm OK, and should he do it a little more firmly? And I focus on my breath in an attempt to simply surrender to all this and neither judge nor compete with the whimpers and heavy breathing and random ecstatic climactic yells I hear from around the room.

And at some stage, the 15 minutes must be up because I feel his hand cup over me as I know it is meant to because this was explained in the orientation, and he checks in with me again.

Then I put my panties and jeans back on and we go our separate ways. He to answer more questions or to OM someone else and I to feel relieved and happy that I've done this. Transported back to the day I lost my virginity.

◞

I don't have the courage to ask someone for a second round. Because it would seem too indulgent? Or because I'd have to ask? My bad, I think, walking back to BART later, when I strike up a conversation with a chiropractor from Sacramento who is delighted that he has learned how to OM and happy that he OMed three women during the day and eager to keep on OMing. Clearly there is something in all of this for at least some men.

◯

And Naomi Wolf, keynote speaker in light of her book, *Vagina: A Cultural History*, has left me with a nugget. Namely, "Don't let a man suck your nipples if you don't want to fall in love with him." (That oxytocin again.) Which comment tickles me in all the right places because if the right man does it, and does it right, indeed, she's right on the button. Although if the wrong man does it, it can have the opposite effect.

And maybe this is a clue to gauging a good man?

And applause for Nicole Daedone. I cannot even imagine what life might have been like, had she been around offering this as an additional meditation practice when I was living at SFZC and being celibate. Who would have thought it possible to connect with a man in this way, no obligation other than to show up and give yourself over? Cultivating mindfulness by being in-the-body present and pleasured? And isn't orgasm the best kind of tonic and lift and better than any bubbly and doesn't it give you a spring in your step and make you feel alive and isn't it good to feed this hungry mouth appropriately?

And doesn't it give a palpable new perspective to the "Do you want food or do you want sex" equation?

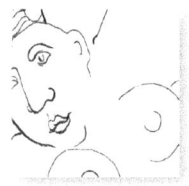

CHAPTER FIFTEEN

ON GIVING GOOD EAR

Six women are having dinner at a Chinese restaurant. At the end of the meal the waiter brings six fortune cookies to the table. Each woman takes one and bites it or breaks it open, as is her way with fortune cookies. For some reason, each small strip of fortune paper is blank.

Woman number one is alarmed. This, she says, is an omen of doom. Nobody must catch a cab home as there is bound to be an accident. The missing fortune, she warns, represents an empty future, which she defines as death.

The second woman laughs ruefully. She says it doesn't mean literal death at all. She says it is a metaphor for her life. "Everything I've done so far amounts to nothing," she laments.

The third woman chides the first two for their doom and gloom. She sees the blank space as a new beginning. "This is the first moment of the rest of my life," she bubbles. "I reckon it's a prompt to start afresh; to create my own good fortune."

The fourth woman interprets it as the sign she has been waiting for. "That's it. It's telling me to end my lousy affair. It's showing me that when I'm with him, my life is as empty as this scrap of paper. And let's face it, empty is empty. How could it be emptier without him?"

The fifth woman says she does not believe in fortune cookies and the reason these ones say nothing is because fortune cookies have nothing to say. Meanwhile, the sixth woman calls the waiter and demands a fortune cookie with a proper message that she can read and understand.

If a group of women are at variance over something as innocuous as a cluster of fortune cookie blanks—and let's face it, give a bunch of us a list of topics, get us going, and most consistent will be our differences—why is it that we listen to generalizations about how we are supposed to think, feel, look and act? Why are so many of us ruled by expectations, stereotypes and demands? Why do we avidly read books and magazine articles on what it is we *really* want—and that even more pervasive self-manipulation: what men want from us?

Why are we constantly searching outside of ourselves for permission?

Does there exist an unacknowledged 13th Commandment that applies specifically to womanhood? Its message: Thou shalt not be thyself.

"What do I want?" is a profound coaching question for many women, more used to being concerned about others than with thinking about—let alone knowing how to identify— their own dreams and desires. Part of knowing what we want is learning to listen. To listen, that is, beneath the external and internal chatter and habits.

"When we are listened to, it creates us, makes us unfold and expand. Ideas actually begin to grow within us and come to life," to quote *If You Want to Write* author Brenda Ueland. "It makes people happy and free when they are listened to," to quote Ueland again. Journaling and memoir writing; *The Artist's Way* author Julia Cameron's morning pages; therapy and coaching; all are great tools for reaching in and learning how to listen to ourselves.

As is meditation.

○

A woman friend goes to the Buddhist Retreat Centre in South Africa. Back from her weekend she tells me: "Well, I can't meditate. My mind thinks all the time. I can't stop it." She has latched on to this story. She has made this her reality. She doesn't want to discuss it. She is not going to try meditating again.

My third or fourth time at the BRC, some time after the bee incident and before I leave for California, I confess to someone: "I've hardly meditated because I keep waking up hung over."

"Meditate on your hangovers," he says.

Touché.

My favorite bumper sticker says: "Don't believe all that you think." This is one of the liberating—and just plain helpful— things you learn when you meditate.

Thing is, if my friend had kept an open mind, she might have gleaned something worthwhile about the nature of this mind. This thinking.

She might have asked the question "Who thinks?" Or "What thinks?" And come to see that "mind thinks."

That the nature of the mind is to think. All the time.

Many thoughts go by like clouds, beyond our awareness. It seems we lock in to certain thoughts that "mind thinks"—and turn them into "I think." Then we make what "I think" very solid, and let what "I think" define, dictate and direct our lives in good or not-so-good ways.

Most of us are simply not aware of this pattern until we spend enough time: just sitting, just breathing, just noticing, naming and letting go—of "thinking," of "story," of "past," of "future"—and coming back to the breath that's breathing us.

And sooner for some and later for others (Suzuki Roshi's fourth type of horse), one becomes more focused and more present. More clear about the nature of the mind. Less commandeered by its whims. More conscious.

◠

"…consciousness is said to be a field, a piece of earth on which every kind of seed is planted. On this field of consciousness are sown the seeds of hope and suffering, the kernel of happiness and sorrow, anger and joy. The quality of our life depends entirely on which seeds we garden and nourish in our consciousness." —former SFZC's Green Gulch Farm head gardener Wendy Johnson from her book Gardening at the Dragon's Gate.

◠

A kind of liberation comes when we see that "mind thinks." That we can go along with selected thoughts if we choose to, and when the thinking serves us. But that if it doesn't, we can change the story.

It's also liberating to know that one story can be as good and as true as the next story; that stories reflecting our truth have a fluidity about them; and that if a person is giving you all manner of reasons for something and making a story solid and "rational" and hard, invariably they've hooked into a story that at some level is helping them make logical sense of their world. Such a story may well represent a fabricated truth. A convenient truth. A truth to avoid cognitive dissonance; not an authentic truth. And all this is likely happening at an unconscious level.

Our way, as humans, is to have our stories. That they're all made up doesn't make them any less real. And it's good to know that we need not be defined by them.

"Until now" is something a coach might say to remind a client that to stay where they are is optional, not required.

And when we get stuck in obsessing over past and future worries, the best thing to do is to get out of the mind, the head, the thinking, and into the realm of the senses. The past is gone, the future might never happen.

We become present in the moment, in the now, when we connect with the physical senses and sensations. When we experience the in-breath and the out-breath. When we become aware of just seeing, just tasting, just touch, just smell, just sound, we access the part of ourselves that knows: what we need to do; what we want. It's also the place of oneness. Of interconnectedness.

At least this is my experience. What I've learned.

⟳

You're making an apple cake. You slice your crisp and juicy Gravenstein into a bowl. So what is it you're slicing? Well, there's the sun and the rain that helped the tree grow; the farmer who tended the tree; the earth with its rich nutrients that supported growth; the harvester who plucked the ripe apple;

the driver who took it to the marketplace; the various people who picked up the apple and maybe put it to their nose and inhaled to capture the fresh smell, before you purchased it to bake and serve to friends who will hopefully relish it. (And at some point return it in a different form to the earth, which maybe we prefer not to think about.)

When I lived at SFZC and was experimenting with food, and my eating habits, and making changes, I did a lot of different things. Like trying to remember to be aware of the field-to-table cycle, not least to counterbalance my usual mindless gobbling. Like eating with chopsticks, also to slow down. And deciding that I could have anything I wanted to eat, the only qualifier being I had to eat it sensually and savor it and "just eat." So, 20 Mars Bars? Sure. Sit down with knife, fork and plate. No distractions. Slice, lift, smell, chew, relish. Each bite like this.

What I found, engaging with food with this seeming abandon, was that first, I would quickly get bored and want to do just about anything other than eat. And second, Mars Bars and many other "forbidden" items, when I gave myself full permission to enjoy them, didn't taste that great beyond the first couple of bites. And if I forced myself to keep going, they became quite gross and I was able to store this new reality in my memory bank.

My consciousness raised by a decision to be "in love" with food and to eat sensually, as in engaging my senses, it became second nature to check labels. Not for calories, but for ingredients. And slowly but surely, because I was being more in my body and mindful, I found I didn't want to eat things with names that were unidentifiable and that didn't sound like food.

I meanwhile browsed food magazines with curiosity, and read about nutrition trends—not from my former "diet" mentality but with an open and receptive mind—and attempted to gauge how my body felt when I ate different foods. Later I got into food writing and culinary travel as a niche. The focus of this immersion being not on what I shouldn't have and didn't want—but on what I found delicious and *did* want.

And all this is about eating well, and nourishment, and nurturing, and quality of life, and vibrant good health, and feeling light and free and sensual and fueled with energy.

With this as the focus, the losing weight part of the equation just happens.

⌒

I meanwhile was also practicing what I had learned during the Zen hospice training—thinking of new nourishments, rewards and treats, dimensions of pleasure and satisfaction. So that when I asked "Do I want food or do I want sex?" I had options to more easily shift and transform those negative old habits around food.

And the thing is, it's all very fluid if we just let it be fluid.

Neuroplasticity means that we can change our brains. We can work with the synapses and create new highways and habits.

The 2004 movie *What the BLEEP Do We Know?!* has a wonderful wedding scene with real people plus little cartoon characters illustrating what goes on with the synapses. It talks about habits and how each time we repeat one, that habit's synapse highway gets stronger and more ingrained. Start doing things a new way, slowly a new synapse pathway builds. Slowly the old solid one begins to atrophy. To lose its grip.

Years back, as a post-grad psych student, I was assigned to teach a class about synapses. My secret weapon was to ask lots of questions and have the bright students give answers. Because it was beyond me then. Words on a page gave me no comprehension. Only when I watched and rewatched this movie did the marrow of the synapse story and the nitty-gritty of neuroplasticity make sense—and a difference to my life.

◯

Somewhere on my journey, it became apparent to me that my compulsive eating, my "being seen" anxiety, my inability to speak out in the world and my depression had all been interlinked. Freedom meant untying the knots, little by little because they were tight—the default synapse highways had been wide and strong—and moving on.

◯

Then, after reading a draft of this book, yet another Helen—this time Australia-based Helen Perry, clinical psychologist, cognitive behavior therapist and co-author of *Experiencing CBT from the Inside Out*—sends me a Facebook message. It's to tell me about a visual analogue Mouth Orgasm (MO) scale she developed when "newly married and new to New Zealand, drowning in the rain, eating my miseries away and in the process gaining 20-plus kilograms."

"You've got me thinking as to what might really have been going on for me," she says.

Perry is no stranger. Once-upon-a-time I was her high school counselor. Since falling down that hole, she got a handle on her eating, relocated to "sunny Brisbane" where she had friends and family, moved on with her life. And forgot about the scale. Till she read my book. "I was thinking, wouldn't this be a nice way to improve one's experience of mindfulness while eating?" she says. "To notice the effects on your pleasure centers."

She points out that a visual analogue scale (VAS) "is by its nature idiosyncratic to each individual and therefore subjective: measuring only *this* person's experience at *this* time, assessed by his or her own anchor points—as established from past experience." So she suggests I think of the most orgasmic thing I've eaten. "That could be your 10. The least orgasmic, your one."

By way of example, Perry recalls her "10" from back then. The temptation that sparked the MO idea. It was a luscious minty ice cream. She relates the sensual experience of eating it. And hey, couldn't one view the anticipation and what she calls "the visual feast"—ogling the dark chocolate flecked with peppermint bits—as foreplay?

This followed by "the weighty feel" of the fat ice cream on a stick between her thumb and forefinger; cracking through the hard, thick chocolate with her teeth; the "hungry mouth and eager tongue" meeting "the cold, gorgeous, creamy ice cream;" the "first shudder of true delight" as the minted swirl of flavor hits her taste buds; the "melting in the mouth, when I have to cry *mmmm.* Followed by a second and third, *mmmm, mmmm, mmmm.*" And then the sugar high that hits "with a warm fuzzy pulsing through my whole body, probably as the endorphins are released."

"The miracle of food," she adds.

I fancy I hear a contented sigh.

A "one" on Perry's scale? "A plain boiled egg. Pleasant and satisfying but no shudders or warm fuzzies afterwards."

Hmm. Wonder how she would have ranked my Scots grandmother's egg flips.

Inspired by Perry's example, and grateful for her gift—she tells me to take what I want from her VAS; to adapt it as I wish—I put it on my mindfulness menu. Try it. Play with it. And find all I need do is ask myself, with interest and curiosity, the obvious question: one through 10, *where* on the MO scale?

I find it "same" but "different" from the "food or sex" buzz phrase. More organic. Makes my mouth water even if there is no food in the picture. Makes me become "in the moment" mindful when food is present: just as Perry said.

At times, when I get into a relationship (seems an appropriate term) with something I consider a treat—into the whole MO experience as in seeing, smelling, texture, flavor, mouth-feel, thinking about how it makes me feel and whether it's what I want to be chowing—I wake up to the fact that I've been seduced by a habit memory and what I'm eating is not so sense-sational after all.

Thinking "Mouth Orgasm" is fun. It's easy. It's instant. Doing it in company feels like a secret decadence. And this simple practice works as a natural barrier to overeating: feeling stuffed being the opposite of orgasmic, sensual or turned on.

I also note that depending on my mood and my hunger, what ranks as a nine on a Monday might switch to a five on

Tuesday, which playfulness and unpredictability keeps the MO game fresh.

On a recent morning at the Buddhist Retreat Center, in South Africa, I've spooned gently bubbling oats from a jumbo pot into a bowl. I've dolloped on natural unsweetened full-cream yoghurt, plopped about a dozen raw almonds on top, added a handful of house-made muesli, some wheat bran and a scattering of linseeds. Eating this in the quiet of the "noble silence" observed at breakfast, I note that on the MO scale, I am giving it a 10. Like a warm and comforting lover, it's satisfying and sublime. Which is not to say a decadent dalliance won't be the object of desire another time, another place.

Part of the joy.

It's like the "do you want food or do you want sex" mantra has come full circle and transformed itself. Thank you Helen P.

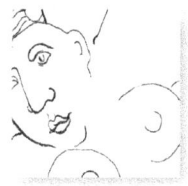

CHAPTER SIXTEEN

LADY MADONNA

I am in Poland and I am suffering.

Self-imposed suffering.

Induced by—a man.

What else?

"To know Poland, you must see Jasna Góra—Black Madonna," Wolfgang, my cousin's husband, says.

I know the image of the Black Madonna from when we swopped holy cards as kids at my Catholic boarding school.

I don't have a clue what Wolfgang is getting at, however, and I don't ask. His English is marginally better than my German, which doesn't go much beyond hand gestures. But whatever Wolfgang and his wife, my cousin, who is Polish, want to show me, I'm in.

We drive on a Saturday morning, from Krakow, initially in the direction of Wrocław.

When I Google later, I learn that Jasna Góra is a monastery in a town called Czestochowa. The Black Madonna, also known as Our Lady of Sorrows, is an icon of the Catholic Virgin Mary housed in a sanctuary there.

○

"Jasna Góra is Poland's Lourdes, Poland's Mecca," Wolfgang says, pointing to a framed picture in the info office where we stop to ask where the loo is after walking from the car park to the imposing monastery complex. The picture shows a massive crowd. "More than 50,000," Wolfgang says. They were, apparently, here for a mass held on the grand concourse when the late Polish Pope John Paul II became Saint John Paul.

"The people—they come for miracles," Wolfgang adds.

"You—Catholic?" I ask Wolfgang, pidgin English style, with hand gestures.

"No," he says.

"Any religion?" I ask.

"Atheist," he says.

○

So there's this guy I've been seeing for going on three years. Do they still have the "it's complicated" relationship button on Facebook? Thing is, it's complicated. I'm divorced, single and unencumbered. He's divorced so therefore single— but encumbered.

Almost enough said. But in brief, this man pursues me till I notice him. Then, till I get curious about him. Then, till I start to like him. Then, till I hop into bed with him. Then, till I get hooked (and not just on hopping into bed with him).

By the time the extent of his encumbrances unfolds, all reason has left the building. He fascinates me, interests me, makes me feel kinda bubbly. And when I ask myself, do I want to ditch him given the encumbrances, which makes very good sense, the answer is no.

Because, hey, it's great to like someone a lot. Even better than being liked by someone (unless the feeling is mutual).

○

This time round, he's been doing what he typically does when we're in different cities: sending me e-mails and photos. Not just of his penis, but that too, which I have read on Facebook is the new norm, although when I share this with a couple of girlfriends, they scoff and say they don't believe a photogenic penis exists.

But this is not about penises.

Although maybe it is, because let's face it, a good one is hard to find. (Or should that read, a hard one is good to find? Delete. Delete.)

So here I've been, in a rental apartment in Krakow for a week while on a kind of mission cum (no, not that kind of cum, Mister) working holiday looking into my Polish roots in an interested but directionless sort of way. And meanwhile, eating and drinking in a more directed way, with the intention of writing travel stories with a focus on food.

He, meanwhile, is in France fixing up an apartment and threatening to cum on my breasts at our next encounter. Funny. But next encounter? When? Those encumbrances again.

He e-mails—about coming to spend time in my bed. I
e-mail—about going to spend time in his.

The e-mails are not just about spending time in bed. They
also talk about drinking wine in cafés, hanging out, giving
ourselves permission and opportunity—just to be together,
which we don't have much chance to do back home. (That
"e" word again.)

Our e-mails are fantasy. We're both in Europe for way too
short a time to logistically make a meeting possible.

The encumbrances (I don't mean to harp, but they are at
the heart of the relationship) both make it (the relationship)
work for me (I feel unencumbered) and not work (he gets close,
I get close, he pulls away, I get encumbered—by pain).

I sometimes wonder how beneficial Zen practice is for
the accommodating and stoic. I tell myself that hurt, when it
comes, is good for my practice. I watch the pain.

I watch how the pain transforms with different thought
patterns.

Sometimes it doesn't transform.

At such times the tears well, even while walking the streets
of Krakow—in awe and wonder, thinking, my god, am I really
here? And isn't it silly to be eating my heart out?

No question, he has hooked deep into my reptilian brain, if
that's the place of inexplicable connection.

Some spark—not his looks, but more how he looked
at me—kindled something in me the first time he literally
snatched at my attention. Greeted me like he knew me, from

the other side of the café I was in, taking my mom for tea and cheesecake.

Something about the encounter disquieted me. Made me feel intruded upon. But interested. It had me ask somebody who he was.

Life force? Energy? Is there some magnetic hook of deep connection? The presence that so visibly had gone out when I saw my father's body, no longer my father, just a body? Do two people inexplicably connect every so often from that space? Am I making up stories? Talking shit?

I can't make sense of our "relationship," but for me, feeling this affinity is a rare thing. I have made a conscious decision that I will not ditch whatever it is that's connecting us unless I have no option.

⟲

Some of these emotions, desires and cravings get stirred up in Krakow, in combination with the welcome overindulgence of being wined, vodkaed and dined on such deliciousness as the plumpest, juiciest smoked carp; sweetbreads I don't like the idea of, but to the palate, tantalizing indulgence; sublime baked cheesecakes; the most delicate melt-in-the-mouth herring; and pierogi, which at their worst can be rubbery, but at their best, especially when stuffed with foraged mushroom, a mouth explosion.

The divine excess of it all swings me back every so often to the "Do I want food or do I want sex?" question.

The one person I'm of a mind to have sex with is only available via e-mail.

And food? It strikes me once again precisely why food can become a sex and comfort and pleasure and relationship substitute. Because let's face it, having a boyfriend, a lover, a significant other, a partner—a rose by any other name—is absolutely no guarantee of good sex, or emotional intimacy, or pleasure and sweet comfort.

But for now, back to the Black Madonna and her shrine. We wander through the overwhelmingly beautiful Jasna Góra church interior. Then continue through to the smaller space, all gold and marble and pillars surreally decorated with crutches and rosaries and what looks like medal memorabilia woven into latticework on the walls. It's already crowded before 10 a.m. I stand in the basilica area, gilded and carved—and there is the distinctive icon herself up in her frame.

I look around. At people gazing at the image. Some with arms outstretched in supplication.

Wolfgang edges in next to me. Points to the left of the altar room.

"You see," he says. "They are in procession. On their knees."

"What?" I don't see. Or understand.

"You must go," he says, nodding, indicating with his head. "Join that line. They walk on knees, round the altar."

Ah, now I see! A single-file thread of people over to my left are "walking" upright on their knees towards the inner sanctum with its high altar. They must be continuing around behind it because I now see people, walking upright on their knees, emerge from behind the altar, to my right.

"Have you done it?" I ask.

"No," he says.

"Why not?" I ask.

He shrugs and shakes his head.

"You not want?" he says.

"No," I reply.

I would feel a hypocrite, for one thing. It would be bloody uncomfortable, is another thing, so you'd need to be doing it for a good reason. I can think of no reason, except to say I'd done it. Like kissing the Blarney Stone, but that was outdoors and more fun.

But—"Can we stay a little while?" I ask.

I just want to be here. To soak in what's going on.

Wolfgang nods. "We have time," he says.

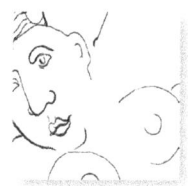

CHAPTER SEVENTEEN

WHAT'S YOUR PLEASURE?

I look round again, at the people. Mostly they are standing, staring at "her." Some are kneeling, hands clasped in prayer.

There is a kneeling person right in front of me.

But no, she's standing. She's just very short.

This wakes me up to a "wow, aren't I lucky" moment.

Something compels me to keep looking; at the faces and at the walls. Those crutches. Symbols of hope for all these men and women with problems. Suffering. Anguish. Hankering. Aching for their lives to be different. The crux of what had the Buddha go sit under the Bodhi tree: to get a handle on the inevitability of death and loss; the "better" scenario of getting old and decrepit; the reality of sickness and a whole range of disappointments; the existential angst of the human condition.

There's a handful of people in wheelchairs but mostly, they are whole and well-dressed. Old people, and young. I try and imagine what they're here for. What they want to add or eliminate. Health issues? Money? Love? Work? Problems involving children? Take a million people, potentially a million tribulations.

Seeing all these mere mortals who've carried their suffering here, and thinking of all the atrocities I read about while swotting up on Poland, plus all I've seen and heard and learned since I arrived—so much more than I already knew about the Holocaust; about Jews and non-Jews massacred before and during World War II; about husbands, fathers, sons, daughters, erased. And that's just looking at the recent history of Poland. Touching the surface. Then what about the nightly world news?

Why, it has me wondering, do we imagine suffering—heartache—is an aberration? A mistake?

Why do we try to deny it? Avoid it? Keep it out of our lives?

What was it Woody Allen said? *Life is full of misery, loneliness and suffering—and it's all over much too soon.* Aches and pains. Loneliness. Old age. Yikes.

I mentally rummage through my friends, thinking about their ups and downs. Hate him one day, love him the next. Losses, rebirths, reinventions. Perspective in each case defining reality. I throw musings of their challenges in with the gilded and marble opulence and those crutches and the prayers, in case the Black Madonna—this woman who must be burned out on people wanting—is listening (gotta hedge your bets). My logical mind says "superstition."

But there's something compelling, to be sure, about living with hope. Like buying a lottery ticket.

○

And hey, I don't mean this to sound dismal.

On the contrary. The vibe here is unaccountably serene. My overwhelming sense is that all of us gathered in this sanctum sanctorum, despite—or ignited by—the challenges, are here having an adventure. It's a balmy October day. There's an effervescent energy in the space. I feel tingly and alive. Is that the faintest aroma of incense or is it my imagination? Along with the serenity there's an absorbing, engulfing radiance. Is it a by-product of hope and belief?

Plus, the artistry is breathtaking. And something about the kneeling procession has tickled my funny bone. Breathing all of this in, becoming one with the surroundings, and connected, I note that I am feeling...the word that comes up is pleasure.

Which makes me think of Darlene Cohen, who stayed across the street from SFZC when I lived there. She had a smile with deep dimples that suffused you like a tonic, and she smiled a lot. When she was made head student for a practice period, which was like a wise role-model position, I was given the job of being her benji, which meant providing support and back-up.

Darlene had been stricken some years previously with rheumatoid arthritis, crippling and excruciating. When she emerged from her apartment block on chilly predawn mornings, I would have been up for maybe 10 minutes. I'd have showered, climbed into my black sweats, put on a little moisturizer and a smear of lipstick, pulled on socks that fitted into my slip-on slip-off zendo sandals and darted across the street to wait for her. She'd have been up for three hours. She'd have spent this time easing her body, her limbs, into the new day; until she had finally limbered up enough to slowly cross the street to take her seat, on a chair, in the meditation hall.

One of Darlene's indelible lessons that I recall, as I stand there, was her story about learning to focus on the moments between the pain. She had come to experience not just relief—but pleasure—in these spaces. Which in turn takes me back to the Zen hospice training program and how we were told to list the things that topped us up and gave us pleasure and to be sure to infuse our lives with them by way of replenishment.

At my cousin's house where I spend three nights before catching the train to Warsaw and flying home, I lie in bed and think about Jasna Góra and all those people suffering and the wars of the ages and the craziness of the world and my piss-in-the-ocean problems that, nonetheless, can be debilitatingly real. I haven't shut myself off in a monastery and I want to live a rich and full life, which is more often than not at odds with comfortable and predictable. Fall in love and risk heartache, walk barefoot on the beach and travel whenever I can, be my own best friend and have other friends who challenge me and make me grow, write my books and ponder the meaning of life. I want to live my own truth, with all the shades of grey of Ansel Adams's zone system, which means there will, at times, be pain.

And I don't understand exactly how it happens, but post-Jasna Góra a new mantra emerges, this one for measuring and living life—and inadvertently adding a huge pleasure principle. And why argue with that?

When I turn on and tune into this new mantra—a three-way dance, in a sense, incorporating adventure, challenge, pleasure—I find I become more in-the-moment present; less in my head, habits and compulsions; and more aware of my body's rhythms. In some ways a similar scenario, though vastly broader than the long-time food or sex yardstick; than the seductive playfulness of the more recent MO scale.

Any time, any place, doing anything, from driving my car to sitting down to a meal to walking into a jazz bar to running in the rain or hiking a country path on a balmy day, I ask myself— and in early days, to get into it, I use little coaching strategies, like wearing a specific bracelet or writing myself sticky notes, to remind me to remember—three questions:

What's the adventure in this?

What is the challenge?

Where's the pleasure?

I find the "trick" is to run through the three steps quickly. No analyzing. The first two parts are head exercises, in a sense, because they involve a quick think. Although in the asking, I find myself becoming present.

The third takes me into my body because what is pleasure other than an experience, a sensation, a feeling? What is pleasure, other than aligning with the senses and via the senses? What is pleasure, other than becoming present, in the moment? To the breath, breathing. To ground beneath feet or butt on seat or my body melding with the contours of another's or my grip on the steering wheel? Unfolding to smells and to tastes and to what I see if I open my eyes, connect and register. To what I hear if I tune in to sound, not to analyze and identify what I'm hearing, but to simply hear sound as sound.

So, one example: I'm at the beach for a swim.

Adventure? Sure thing. Here I am in the Indian Ocean, swimming with unknown sea creatures. What might happen in the next few minutes? Who knows. Curiosity and not knowing make for adventure.

Challenge? A challenge can be negative or it can be positive. Today, in this ocean, it's positive. There are tides. I must watch for waves. I must keep afloat and aware. But conditions are gentle.

Pleasure? Aha. I say the word, I feel the pleasure: like a whispering flutter of oxytocin. Of floating. Of the water buoying me up. Of the saltiness when I lick my lips. Of the sun, warming every part of me that's not submerged. The morning—golden. I'm having an in-the-body experience. It's got me out of my head. Blissful pleasure. Not doing anything special. Just awareness. A "being in the moment" place.

I find none of this is about seeking pleasure. It's not about doing anything differently.

It's simply about awareness. Noticing. Becoming mindful— pretty effortlessly.

The "pleasure" quotient, like magic, when I say the word, shifts me out of my head into my body. Connecting with "pleasure" pulls me into the present. And there is pleasure in the present.

And I find this triad works in good times and in not so good times because it stops me from getting caught in my stories.

And I can thank the man with encumbrances and Jasna Góra and my cousin's husband and Darlene Cohen and an endless list of tangible and intangible, remembered and long-forgotten, influences for this triple-treasure template that bubbles up and gives me a new touchstone for living with heightened pleasure: by highlighting pleasure. If you try it and it works for you, use it with my pleasure.

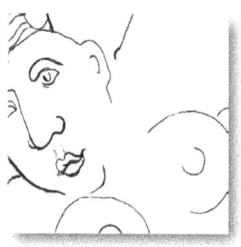

CHAPTER EIGHTEEN

AFTERGLOW:
A Visualization

Breathe. Suspend reality. Visualize this.

You're walking, walking, walking—down a street in your favorite city. It could be London, Paris, Cape Town, Krakow, Buenos Aires, Berlin.

I'll make mine San Francisco.

You're walking, but not just "anyhow" walking. Whatever your age and regardless of your attitude to physical activity, or to your body's good points, or to any parts you're inclined to criticize, you're "out there" walking, feeling alive, energized, ebullient—and sensual, as in tuned in to your senses.

You're fully embracing, experiencing and relishing your energy.

You feel your breath as it flows in and then out again, in and then out, deeply and rhythmically; you're aware of your muscles, strong and flexible, carrying you; aware of your body, which feels supple, lithe and limber.

Your eyes scan the faces, the façades of buildings, the colors of the day and how the light reflects. Your ears are attuned to the sounds of the traffic, the people-noises, and all that's alive around you. Focused on your body, your energy, your spunkiness—and alert to the physical sensations—you've moved out of your head and into a "not thinking" space.

Here and now, in this moment, you are just "being."

You have a strong awareness that you feel safe: supported by the ground, which you're conscious is holding you, and by a universe you know you can trust.

And now, as you keep walking, fluidly and at an energetic pace, embracing your body, you step…right out of your clothes. Stay with me on this journey; no "buts" allowed. Any pooh-poohing or self-criticism, breathe in deeply; breathe out.

Consciously let it go and purposefully continue your zippy hike, in your mind's eye stripped naked, not just enjoying your body and your energy but *loving* it. On a high, inhibitions dropped, delighting in the sensations you discern.

Now, as you keep walking, you become aware that what you were experiencing as robust and invigorating is growing more intense and you begin to luxuriate in an awesome sense of freedom and in-the-body alertness. You note that you feel self-contained and amused and playfully sexy. You're flaunting it, whatever "it" is. But just for yourself. Because this is for you. You're safe in your private nakedness.

As you grow more comfortable and get more of a kick out of your little game, you start making eye contact with people you pass in the street. How nurturing and abundant the world is from this place.

You smile. They smile back. You're wordlessly inviting the people you engage with to "Look at me. See me. Admire me."

This is about your energy. Your being. Your appreciation of you. You're allowing them to share it with you. You breathe in their appreciation as they *really* see your essence and know you for what is your unadulterated, unique, natural, energized, sensual and playful self.

In turn, looking at those you make eye contact with, you see their energy, sensuality, life force and goodwill and you admire them back; embrace them. You notice how you can mentally jump inside the skin of any one of them and effectively "become" them: a most powerful experience of oneness. No judgment. Just energy and the flow of life.

Feeling delighted now, caught up as you are in this pleasure-filled experience of celebratory sashaying, you become appreciatively aware that you got out of bed this morning with a similar mix of zest and joie de vivre. How good it is living in a liberated place where it's totally OK to be "you," vulnerable parts included.

You're happy to embrace the philosophy of perfect just as you are[1] (with, here and there, a little room for nurturing self-improvement). This notion connects you, in a tangible way, to that deep-knowing place of wisdom, intuition and lightness of being: open to you any time you connect with your breath and switch off the mental chatter that can be so loud, compelling and taxing.

You breathe in gratitude for having learned, when anxieties niggle, that "this too will pass." On those now-rare days when you wake pre-dawn—rational mind stifled by sleep, defenses down and in that dark-night-of-the-soul space, unguarded and open to fear and worries—you know to focus your attention on the swinging door moving in, as you inhale; out, as you exhale.[2] You know to connect with your breath, let it breathe you, and that worries reconfigure.

You know to scribble down or mentally conjure up different ways to look at what's bugging you.

You've learned how delicious life can be when you feel gratitude for big things and small things and especially for how good you feel about your body, for all that it gives you by way of service and pleasure.

Related to this, how turned on you feel about yourself and your life when you tune in to the sexual and sensual spark that ignited when you switched to nourishing, nurturing and pleasuring yourself with all you eat and drink, starting with your first cup of coffee or tea, strawberry-mango smoothie, juiced beetroot, apple and carrot blend or morning decadence. Whatever your body asks you for; scope unrestricted and unlimited.

You love the effervescence—the bouncy "I'm desirable" self-affirmation—that has infused you since you developed a pleasure-centered abundance-focused relationship with food and from this kick-off point, with yourself, others, and the world. You love the liberation that came with the illumination of some sticky black holes. With seeing the interconnection between the two hungry mouths. With turning on and tuning in to your body in large part by feeding it well with yummy things savored, relished and appreciated.

And how you've added oodles of pleasure to moments you would not have thought of as pleasure-filled by regularly tapping in and rating what you're doing and who you're being in terms of adventure, challenge and pleasure; this bringing you back more and more easily and regularly to being present, in the moment, aware of "the now."

It's exhilarating to know you're a magnet for good things when you feel good. And that feeling rich is about being rich in friendships, health, well-being and the relationship you have with life, the people in your life, your work, with yourself and your world.

As you continue on your free-spirited hike through the city, you're aware that this is a liberating place. A place of choice and possibility.

You breathe in life. You breathe in the world.

Life is good.

○

REFERENCES

1 Shunryu Suzuki Roshi: *Zen Mind, Beginner's Mind*.
2 Shunryu Suzuki Roshi: *Zen Mind, Beginner's Mind*: "What we call 'I' is just a swinging door which moves when we inhale and when we exhale."

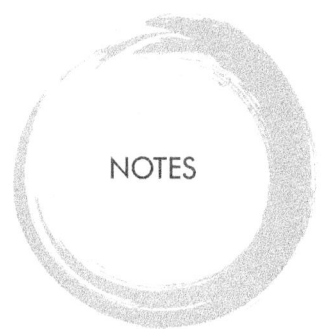

NOTES

ABOUT THE AUTHOR

Wanda Hennig worked as a journalist and editor on newspapers and as bureau chief for the South African edition of Cosmopolitan magazine before moving to California. In *Cravings*, she draws on her psychology and life coaching training and experience and long-time Zen practice. She is an award-winning travel and culinary travel writer. Many of the insights shared in this memoir-cum-self-help were gleaned while traveling: in and around South Africa, the San Francisco Bay Area, Poland, Paris, Pocatello, Salt Lake City and elsewhere.

wandahennig.com
Facebook: wanda.hennig
Instagram: @wanda_hennig
Twitter: @wandahennig

Lightning Source UK Ltd.
Milton Keynes UK
UKHW021436210119
335940UK00006B/663/P